Power and Nursing Practice

Sociology and Nursing Practice Series

Margaret Miers
Gender Issues and Nursing Practice

Sam Porter
Social Theory and Nursing Practice

Geoff Wilkinson and Margaret Miers (eds)
Power and Nursing Practice

Sociology and Nursing Practice Series
Series Standing Order
ISBN 0–333–69329–9
(outside North America only)

You can receive future titles in this series as they are published by placing a standing order. Please contact your bookseller or, in the case of difficulty, write to us at the address below with your name and address, the title of the series and the ISBN quoted above.

Customer Services Department, Macmillan Distribution Ltd
Houndmills, Basingstoke, Hampshire RG21 6XS, England

Power and Nursing Practice

Edited by

Geoff Wilkinson and Margaret Miers

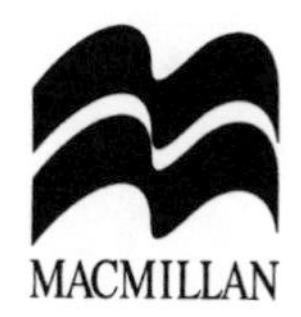

First published 1999 by
MACMILLAN PRESS LTD
Houndmills, Basingstoke, Hampshire RG21 6XS
and London
Companies and representatives throughout the world

ISBN 0–333–69196–2 paperback

A catalogue record for this book is available from the British Library.

This book is printed on paper suitable for recycling and made from fully managed and sustained forest sources.

10 9 8 7 6 5 4 3 2 1
08 07 06 05 04 03 02 01 00 99

Editing and origination by
Aardvark Editorial, Mendham, Suffolk

Printed in Malaysia

Contents

Series Editors' Preface

It is widely accepted that because sociology can provide nurses with valuable and pertinent insights, it should be a constituent part of nursing's knowledge base. To take but a few substantive examples, sociology can help nurses to understand the causes and distribution of ill health, the experience of illness, the dynamics of health care encounters and the limitations and possibilities of professional care. Equally importantly, sociology's emphasis on critical reflection can encourage nurses to be more questioning and self-aware, thus helping them to provide flexible, non-discriminatory, client-centred care.

Unfortunately, while the aspiration of integrating sociology into nursing knowledge is easy enough to state in theory, in practice their relationship has not been as productive as some might have hoped. Notwithstanding a number of works that have successfully applied sociological tools to nursing problems, there remains a gulf between the two disciplines, which has led some to question the utility of the relationship.

On the one hand, sociologists, while taking an interest in nursing's occupational position, have not paid great attention to the actual work that nurses do. This is partially the result of the limitations of sociological surveillance. Nurses work in confidential, private and intimate settings with their clients, and sociologists' access to such settings is necessarily restricted. Moreover, nurses find it difficult to talk about their work, except to other nurses. As a result, core issues pertaining to nursing have been less than thoroughly treated in the sociological literature. There is thus a disjunction between what nurses require from sociology and what sociologists can provide.

On the other hand, nurses are on equally uncertain ground when they attempt to use sociology themselves. Nurses are often reliant on carefully simplified introductory texts, which, because of their broad remit, are often unable to provide an in-depth understanding of sociological insights. Nor is it simply a matter of knowledge; there are tensions between the outlooks of nursing and of sociology. Because nursing work involves individual interactions, it is not surprising that when nurses turn to sociology, they turn to those elements that concentrate on microsocial interaction. While this is useful in so far as it goes, it does not provide nurses with knowledge of the restraints and enablements imposed upon individual actions by social structures.

The aim of the *Sociology and Nursing Practice* series is to bridge these gaps between the disciplines. The authors of the series are nurses or teachers of nurses and therefore have an intimate understanding of nursing work and an appreciation of the importance of individualised nursing care. Yet at the same time, they are committed to a sociological outlook that asserts the salience of wider social forces to the work of nurses. The texts apply sociological theories and concepts to practical aspects of nursing. They explore nursing care as part of the social world, showing how different approaches to understanding the relationship between the individual and society have implications for nursing practice. By concentrating on a specific aspect of sociology or nursing, each book is able to provide the reader with a deeper knowledge of those aspects of sociology most pertinent to their own area of work or study. We hope that the series will encourage nurses to analyse critically their practice and profession, and to develop their own contribution to health care.

Margaret Miers, Sam Porter and Geoff Wilkinson

Acknowledgements

This book, and the series of which it is a part, owes much to the support of many of those involved in nurse education. We are grateful to our colleagues in the former Sociology Theme Team, Avon and Gloucestershire College of Health 1991–96, many of whom have contributed to this volume. We are indebted to Sam Porter, co-editor of the *Sociology and Nursing Practice* series, for making the series a reality. It was Margaret O'Gorman's interest in this book and the series that gave us initial encouragement. Richenda Milton-Thompson's patient support throughout our hesitant progress has been exemplary. We owe thanks to our families, Ruth, Tom and Matthew and David, John and Anne. We are grateful for their tolerance. Thanks, too, to Chris Pickering for his patient assistance.

Geoff Wilkinson and Margaret Miers

Notes on Contributors

Anthony Fraher RMN, RGN, CertEd(FE), DN(Lond), MSc is a Senior Lecturer in the School of Mental Health and Learning Disability at the University of the West of England, Bristol. Particular interests are around mental health provision for elderly people and those from ethnic minority backgrounds, with a specific focus on advocacy and empowerment.

Jane Godfrey MA, RGN, RMN, CertEd(FE), RNT was formerly a Senior Lecturer in the Faculty of Health and Social Care, University of the West of England, Bristol. She is currently employed as a practitioner in renal care. Her special interests revolve around the experience of health care by gay and lesbian people.

Matthew Godsell BA(Hons), MEd, PGGE(FE), RNT, RNMH is a Senior Lecturer at the Faculty of Health and Social Care, University of the West of England, Bristol. His interests are social policy and research. He is studying the history of services for people with learning disabilities for a PhD at the University of Bristol.

Michel Limpinnian RGN, RMN, DN(Lond), RCNT, RNT, MSc is a Senior Lecturer in the School of Mental Health and Learning Disability at the Faculty of Health and Social Care, University of the West of England, Bristol. His particular interests are sociology, social policy and complementary therapies, especially in relation to people with mental health needs.

Gillian Mowforth BEd(Hons), MSc, RGN, CertEd(FE), DipN(Lon) is a Senior Lecturer in the School of Adult Nursing Studies, the Faculty of Health and Social Care, University of the West of England, Bristol. She has worked extensively in the field of adult nursing, especially in the area of critical care. Her special interests are how sociology and social policy impacts and can illuminate nursing by assisting in its critical evaluation.

Margaret Miers BA, MSc, PhD, RGN, PGCert(HE) is a Senior Lecturer, Health Studies, in the Faculty of Health and Social Care, University of the West of England, Bristol. She has worked as a lecturer in sociology with special interests in health care, cultural studies and nurse education. Her health care experience includes research into health promotion and primary care and five years working as a nurse, and in a combined research/practitioner role in breast care.

Sam Porter RN, DipN, PhD is a Senior Lecturer in Sociology, Department of Sociology and Social Policy, Queen's University, Belfast. He has eight years' experience as a clinical nurse, and now teaches social theory and the sociology of health. He publishes in both sociological and nursing journals and is the author of *Social Theory and Nursing Practice* in this series.

Drew Thomas BA(Hons), RGN, PGCE(FE), Dip HE(DN) is a part-time Senior Lecturer in the School of Community Nursing, Faculty of Health and Social Care, University of the West of England, Bristol, while also working as a district nurse for the United Bristol Healthcare Trust. His main interest is in the arena of community nursing, particularly in relation to health and social issues affecting older people.

Geoff Wilkinson RMN, RNMH, RCNT, RNT, CertEd(FE), MSc is a Senior Lecturer in the School of Mental Health and Learning Disability, Faculty of Health and Social Care, University of the West of England, Bristol. His main interests are health and social care provision for people with a learning disability/difficulty and social policies pertinent to them.

Introduction

Nursing is not a powerful profession. Nursing as an activity takes place in a context of power differentials and social inequalities. Nursing's form and relationships have evolved over time, and what we imagine nursing to be today is the consequence of varied and complex interactions in a number of spheres and at a number of levels. Its current location in a centrally administered welfare system exposes it to the vagaries of political will and economic change, which has a direct effect on the work nurses do and where and with whom they do it. This book derives from concern that student nurses are rarely introduced to ways of analysing power that derive from social theories despite a proliferation of articles on and interest in nurses' role in the empowerment of those for whom they care.

Nursing is not an activity that occurs in a vacuum. At work, nurses enter into relationships that span a wide sphere. There are power dynamics involved in relationships within nursing, often based on official hierarchies and on deeper, less immediately visible, social structures such as age, gender, ethnicity and ability. Power is involved in interactions with users of health services, be they constructed as patients, clients or service users, just as there is power at work in the construction and reconstruction of these labels, which, in turn, bring with them different care and treatment connotations. The construction of care and treatment regimes and settings is in itself evidence of power, in this instance the power that comes with knowledge, skills and attitudes: those of the professional practitioner.

Neither do nurses work in isolation from other occupational and professional groups, many of whom are also competing for, or maintaining, professional status and the rewards that come with it. Each of these groups works with its own model of health and illness; not all of the models necessarily happily co-exist, yet they are frequently simultaneously applied to the same territory – the body or mind of the patient/client. The patient herself can become the site of inter-professional rivalry and conflict, becoming simultaneously objectified and subjectified. These claims to the body and mind are made on a number of grounds ranging from medical to managerial. Nurses may find themselves in the role of negotiator or mediator in this contested space.

Relationships can stretch beyond the arena of health services. Many patients/clients have needs other than those directly related to 'illness'. Nurses will frequently become involved with social care agencies and their representatives. When the current structures of the mixed economy of care and quasi-markets (LeGrand and Bartlett 1993) and future possibilities for health action zones (DoH 1997a) are taken into consideration, the range of service providers expands to include, for example, voluntary and charitable bodies, community groups and workers, and housing associations. The potential for different ideologies to emerge and meet is again evident.

The foregoing may indeed be a pessimistic account, assuming as it does the existence of rivalry, struggle and conflict. The social world and the world of health care are perhaps grounded much more in consensus than has been indicated. Whichever the case may be, an understanding of sociological theories of power may be of help to nurses attempting to work within the changing structures, discourses and relationships of health care policy and practice. Such an understanding has certainly helped the contributors to this text as we worked together introducing students to social science-based approaches to understanding health and health care. Varied conceptual frameworks helped us explore the complexity of the changes we were (and are) experiencing in nurse education. Our own feelings of disempowerment as we sought to maintain support for our students despite declining resources and increased productivity enhanced our concern to explore approaches to understanding power. In our teaching, we selected theories of power and authority (notably those of Lukes 1974, and Weber 1948), chosen on the basis of what made most sense to us, theories that might help nurses to identify and work effectively within the power dynamics involved in policy changes and in professional practice (Aust *et al.* 1997).

This book is structured in four main parts. Part I concentrates on the conceptual analysis of power and professional power, drawing on sociological ideas and literature. Parts II, III and IV concentrate on exploring power issues in nursing, often illustrating the relevance of the analytical approaches introduced in

Chapters 1 and 2. The chapters in Part II look at power issues between nurses and within the nursing profession. Mowforth explores the relationship between gender, power and nursing, (Chapter 3) and the subtle effects of élitism within the profession (Chapter 4), arguing, among other things, that it can be useful to see nurses as an oppressed group. Miers (Chapter 5) looks at the positive and negative consequences of hierarchical structures and the qualities of leaders in care settings.

Part III looks at nurses in the health care team, focusing specifically on nurses as health care workers (Chapter 6), nurses' relationships with doctors (Chapter 7) and power issues in community care (Chapter 8). The importance of understanding labour market processes when trying to understand nurses' relatively subordinate position as workers is central to Miers' analysis of nurses' work. Porter also identifies changing patterns of work organisation as important in attempting to understand changing work relationships between nurses and doctors. The possibilities of nurses developing their roles and improving their status within health and social care teams are examined through an explicitly Foucauldian analysis of power in Chapter 8. Understanding professional models of care as discourses that can discipline or enable professionals, colleagues, teams and clients may help nurses to develop new roles in primary health and community care's contested space.

Nurses' relationships with clients are considered in the chapters in Part IV. These chapters concern a variety of settings and specialisms, and look at changes in health care practice that have developed through a concern to give service users more choice and more control. Chapters 10 and 14 both look at the movement of clients into the community, with some pessimism. Chapter 11 looks at changes in the practice of administering medicines as a means of giving power back to children and their carers. Chapter 13 explores issues in relation to involving clients in decision making. Both these chapters seek to identify whether and how nurses might be able to 'make a difference' through their care, focusing on Giddens' (1984) analysis of power in structuration theory, on Lukes' (1974) analysis of three faces of power and on the discursive power of knowledge and practices (see Chapter 1). Chapters 9 and 12 seek to develop readers' understanding of the inequalities faced by older persons, gay men and lesbians as service users, and the structural origins of discriminatory practices. Thomas (Chapter 9) and Godfrey (Chapter 12) are optimistic about nurses' potential to care within a philosophy of anti-discriminatory practice. Godsell (Chapter 14) and Fraher and Limpinnian (Chapter 10) see changes in our understanding of professional authority as necessary for the empowerment of users of mental health and learning disabilities services.

One of the aims of the *Sociology and Nursing Practice* series is to encourage the interchange of ideas between nurses and sociologists. Whereas all contributors to this volume are nurses, the authors have varied responsibilities for teaching sociology to health care practitioners and other students. Some authors have drawn heavily on the sociological literature about power and about nursing, while others have focused on exploring and explaining the effect of the social context on power dynamics in health care, drawing on policy and health literature as much as on sociology. The conclusion reflects on the potential of the interchange for nurses, sociologists and health care practice.

PART I

Understanding power

1 Theories of power

Geoff Wilkinson

Introduction

Power is an essentially contested concept. There is a range and diversity of interpretations of what is meant by power. This chapter will outline the main arguments from a variety of perspectives and identify their main elements.

Theories of power

It is usual to distinguish two forms of power: authority and coercion. When the exercise of power is accepted as legitimate by those upon whom it is exercised, it is regarded as authority. However, when its exercise is not accepted as legitimate, it is seen as coercion. It is, of course, not so clear cut, since it can be argued that both are ultimately based on the use of physical force. The nature of nursing care places a responsibility on nurses to reflect on the difference as well as the close relationship between authority and coercion.

Weberian approach

Giddens (1971) describes Weber's definition of power as 'the probability that an actor will be able to realise his own objectives even against opposition from others with whom he is in a social relationship' (p. 156). In Haralambos and Holborn (1991), the translation is slightly different. Power is 'the chance of a man or a number of men to realise their own will in a communal action even against the resistance of others who are participating in the action' (pp. 117–18). Putting aside the inherent sexism, Weber is arguing that power is evident when one party gets his or her own way, despite opposition. Thus power is evident when one party achieves its will over another. This may occur through coercion or submission to domination, but more frequently through authority.

Weber (1948) also addressed the issue of authority and identified three ideal types: charismatic authority, in which an individual's personal qualities are such that they engender admiration and loyalty (he cites Alexander the Great, Napoleon Bonaparte and Jesus Christ as examples); traditional authority, which is based on the 'rightness' of established practices and loyalty, and is grounded in obligation (the feudal system serves as an illustration); and rational-legal authority, which is based on impersonal rules frequently supported by a legal framework (the legal and military systems are examples, as is bureaucracy). Weber accepts that there are no perfect examples of these ideal types. Chapter 11 makes use of Weber's types of authority to look at power issues in caring for children. Whereas the traditional authority of doctors may inhibit the acceptance of nurses' autonomy in professional practice, rational-legal authority, through specialist education for children's nursing, helps to promote the power of registered nurses.

Inherent in Weber's definition is the assumption that power is held only at the expense of others because there is only so much to go around. This view of power has been described as the 'constant sum' concept of power. The other significant point that Weber makes is that those who hold power use it to their own ends.

Radical approaches

Lukes (1974) suggests that Weber's analysis is too narrow and postulates, in a radical argument, that power has three dimensions, or faces. The first face is in general agreement with Weber in that power can be detected when issues are settled in favour of one group over another. Lukes goes further and, drawing on the work of Bachrach and Baratz (1962); makes a case for a second face of power, arguing that power can be detected in non-decision making. Power can be exercised to keep items off the agenda and is therefore used to keep decision making in the arena controlled by the powerful. Thus power is used to limit discussion, the range of alternative actions available is constrained, and decisions taken therefore remain under the control of the powerful actors such as the professionals and managers involved in decision making in health care.

Lukes (1974) then offers a third dimension or face, arguing that powerful individuals and groups are able to manipulate the wishes and desires of others who can be persuaded to accept things that may even be harmful to them. From this point of view, he would be in general agreement with a feminist stance that exposes the damaging effects of patriarchy on women and children. Expectations concerning women's dress, for example, may serve the interests of men who have financial control over the fashion market. Images of nurses as sexy, available and desirable can offer nurses the attraction of attention while denying them a role in health care decision making. The Marxist analysis of the harm done to the proletariat by the forms of organisation of capitalist societies, through the development of false class consciousness, is another example that supports the proposed third face.

Workers may view increased material wealth as a symbol of higher class status, failing to recognise continuing exploitation under relationships of private property. Illich's (1977) notion of cultural iatrogenesis, whereby cultural acceptance of medicine's role leads to dependency on professional care, is a health-related example of the third face.

The theories examined so far accept two important points in Weber's definition: first, that power is held at the expense of others (the 'constant sum' concept); and second, those who hold power use it in their own interests.

Functionalist approaches

Functionalists would generally disagree with both of these propositions. Functionalism suggests that social actions and institutions are capable of being understood by identifying their function, that is, their contribution to the maintenance of the social system as a whole. Power is a resource held by individuals and groups in relation to the importance of their activities to society's collective goals. Parsons (1951) rejects the constant sum concept, seeing power as a 'generalised resource' possessed by the whole society. He proposes an alternative 'variable sum' concept, arguing that power increases in a society the more that a society achieves its desired communal ends. Increased productivity, for example, will create greater profits, leading to a higher standard of living, so everybody is more powerful. This equation can, of course, work the other way, and the effects of reduced productivity would ultimately lead to loss of power to that society and its members. It is for this reason that Parson calls it the 'variable sum' concept. In a period of recession and consequent political responses to contain NHS costs, for example, the enhancement of the managers' role in controlling costs, the reduction in the number of qualified nurses and the rise in the number of health care assistants can be seen as part of an overall reduction in the power of the professionals most closely associated with the NHS – doctors and nurses.

Parsons applies the variable sum concept to political power in a democracy, suggesting that political power is invested in the ballot box. At an election, politicians gain or lose votes depending upon how successful, or otherwise, they have been in achieving the ends of the electorate. Parsons is criticised on the grounds of offering a naïve, uncritical and apologist description that has sociologically rationalised power holders' own justification for holding power and also for failing to recognise the exercise of power to further the interests of some at a cost to others.

Pluralist approaches

Pluralists (see Chapter 4) also offer explanations of the distribution of power in Western democratic societies. There are two schools of pluralist thought: classical and élite. The latter emerged in response to criticisms of the former.

Classical pluralism sees Western democracies as the most advanced forms of government yet devised and holds that the exercise of power by the state is legitimate because governments act in accord with the wishes of the population from whom political power is ultimately derived. In this, they are in general accord with Parsons. However, they differ in a number of ways. The 'variable sum' concept is rejected in favour of Weber's constant sum; the notion of political representation based on a social value consensus is not accepted, and, following from this, the role of the state is perceived as one of being an honest broker between a range of competing interests. The state is not seen as able to represent consensus since pluralists deny that value consensus can exist. Government is the business of compromise and mediation between different interests.

Criticisms of classical pluralism mirror, to some extent, those applied to functionalist approaches. By not acknowledging the possibility of the second and third faces, pluralists maintain the illusion of power as a widely distributed social resource, confirming a belief in democratic systems while simultaneously concealing the real bases of power from scrutiny and thereby protecting the powerful. Concealment of the third dimension creates a 'false class consciousness', which disguises the real interests of the population from itself, perpetuating the political system in the interests of the powerful. As a consequence of these and other criticisms, classical pluralism was reappraised and re-emerged as élite pluralism. Any pluralist standpoint on the nature and development of the NHS in Britain would acknowledge that, however popular the idea of a service free at the point of use, the actual form of service adopted is always a compromise between different interests, notably those of consultants, GPs, the government, health service managers and (considerably less importantly) unions and professional organisations representing other health care workers.

Elite pluralism is similar to its precursor, classical pluralism, in that it sees Western government as democratic and therefore superior to pre-existing forms, and believes that power is widely dispersed in the population and that government is essentially the process of compromise. It parts company in a number of significant ways, particularly in its analysis of the distribution of power, which it concludes is held unequally. It accepts that well-organised groups can exert control over the agenda, allowing élites to be the main decision makers in society. (Elitism in nursing is discussed in Chapter 4.) It thus incorporates the second face of power and also acknowledges the possibility of some not being represented, albeit temporarily, and others not being politically active. While this may be regarded as progress in our understanding of power in society, there are still a number of faults with the arguments. The main fracture is that, in accepting the possibility of democracies as faulty, the underlying tenet of classical pluralism, that power is widespread in society, is exposed to doubt. In addition to this, the uncritical acceptance of élites as essentially functional to society does not allow for the consideration of their *use* of power, particularly in relation to furthering their own ends. Finally, the existence of the third face of power and the possibility of shaping desires is not entertained.

It can be argued that, with the exception of Lukes (1974) and Weber, these structural approaches to the analysis of power have been revealed as essentially functionalist. Other structural approaches, particularly Marxist/conflict approaches, should not be ignored. On the whole, these perspectives adopt a very different stance from those preceding them and, as will be demonstrated, can be numbered among the most trenchant critics of consensus approaches.

Marxist approaches

In general, Marxist/conflict approaches see power as being concentrated in the hands of minorities and used by them to further their own interests. The different interests of different groups are among the sources of potential conflict. The assumption of power being independently invested in the state is disputed; instead, it arises specifically from control over, or access to, economic resources. Marxists argue that the exercise of this power is essentially coercive because the subject class, the proletariat, submits to a situation that is against its best interests. The power of the bourgeoisie extends from the infrastructure, the economic base, and penetrates the superstructure, which includes politics and culture. Consequently, the state reflects the distribution of power in society. In this account, it is inevitable that the decisions of the state will favour the ruling class to the detriment of the general population.

On the face of it, this is quite straightforward but, inevitably, writers from this background find themselves in conflict. To illustrate this, the contrasting positions of Miliband (1969) and Poulantzas (1978), both writing in the Marxist tradition, will be described.

Miliband proposes an instrumentalist view, that is, a view that regards the state as an instrument (or tool) of the bourgeoisie. He argues that power is derived from wealth. The instrument of the state is used to preserve economic dominance, maintain political power and stabilise capitalist society in the interests of the economically powerful, that is, the bourgeoisie. This, in Miliband's analysis, is achieved because the state is run by a number of élites that act together to serve the interests of capital and private property. As evidence to support this contention, Miliband offers the following: élite positions are held by the bourgeoisie, which is bound together by kinship, educational background and interests; many originate from upper- or upper-middle class families; the majority attended public schools and Oxbridge; thus all of them have been socialised into the ruling class. Miliband argues that socially mobile members of élites who have gained access from the working class have adopted the values, mores and manners of the bourgeoisie. Governmental power is accepted by the proletariat because the bourgeoisie are able to manipulate their wishes and desires through processes such as advertising, which promotes the view that happiness derives from the material benefits of economic success. Adverts for medicines to relieve pain, indigestion, coughs and colds are promoting pharmaceutical interests rather than the health and welfare of the population. The third face of power perpetuates the *status quo*.

In this analysis, instrumental individual human agency shapes and moulds the superstructure to the benefit of the powerful. Poulantzas (1978) offers a different perspective, one that minimises the effects of agency and re-emphasises the importance of social structure. In Poulantzas' view, the state is vital to the stability and maintenance of capitalism and *automatically* serves ruling class interests. Elites are irrelevant to his analysis because the capitalist system in itself is sufficient to ensure that the interests of the ruling class are served. This also has the benefit of making the state and the bourgeoisie appear relatively autonomous. Neither does Poulantzas agree with Miliband about the mechanisms of legitimation, although he acknowledges the vital role of aspects of culture. In Poulantzas' scenario, legitimation is tied directly to the state via its control of the repressive and ideological state apparatus. The former is related to coercive power and includes the government, armed forces, police, courts and tribunals. The latter includes religion, political parties, unions, schools, media and the family, and is more concerned with the manipulation of beliefs and values. Political ideologies such as liberalism, individualism and socialism can all affect the development of health service policy and thereby affect nursing. The dominance of biomedical models of health and health care can also play a role in social control and in the control of nursing.

Miliband responds to this view of legitimation by accusing Poulantzas of 'structural super-determinism', arguing that the infrastructure is not sufficiently powerful to determine all human behaviour and that there is little evidence to support this assertion. Both Miliband and Poulantzas, however, largely agree that it is in the power of the infrastructure to mould the superstructure; only the mechanisms are disputed.

Neo-Marxist approaches

Gramsci (1971), while not disputing the importance of the infrastructure, at least as the background against which social relations are acted out, denied its significance in relation to the superstructure. He also differed from Marx in his view of the state, arguing that it is composed of a dominant class constituted through compromise and negotiation rather than in terms of institutions. He was also dubious about the power of economic determinism, to the point of rejecting it.

In Gramsci's analysis, the superstructure is composed of two elements – political and civil society. Political society holds the monopoly on the use of coercive mechanisms such as the army, police and judicial system, whereas civil society is primarily institutions such as the Church, trades unions and political parties. The state is defined in terms of the activities of dominant classes rather than in terms of institutions created for them. Central to Gramsci's description of power is the idea of hegemony, which denotes general and intellectual dominance and implies an acceptance of dominant ideas. Dominant groups gain control through gaining active acceptance and approval of their ideas by articulating shared interests between dominated and dominating groups. The ruling class is prepared to compromise, both in its own interests and in those of the subordinate class. Hegemony is essentially power gained through the generation and acceptance of ideas by the ruling groups and the acceptance of these ideas by the ruled as a compromise to maintain the stability of the social order.

In some ways, hegemony reflects both Marxist analysis of the process of generating false class consciousness and Lukes' (1974) third face of power. The force of ideas is recognised, but its origins are located elsewhere (that is, in shared rather than opposed interests) and its consequences are different (a negotiated consensus based on accepting the idea of minimising rather than maximising exploitation). Inherent in all of this is the recognition that even similarly placed groups in society do not necessarily share the same interests. It would be possible to analyse the changing health policy context as a search for hegemonic ideas that could unite health care workers and service users, reaffirming support for the NHS (itself a hegemonic idea) while allowing it to change. The 1997 White Paper *The New NHS* (DoH 1997a) articulates a new model for a new century, 'based on partnership and driven by performance', retaining the separation between planning and provision and developing primary care through allocating resources to primary care groups comprising GPs and community nurses. Primary care groups can be seen as a reformulation of the idea of GP fundholding, an aspect of the internal market that eventually attracted significant support. In the process of changing policies and ideas, the government is explicitly attempting to retain the NHS as a national service that has public confidence, recognising its role as a hegemonic idea in British culture.

Structuration

The arguments presented so far have, in general, emphasised the primacy of structures over agency, although Miliband and Gramsci's ideas moved away from super-determinism. To some extent, the Weberian standpoint, seeing power as the probability that an actor will be able to realise objectives, has re-emerged in Giddens' structuration theory, an analysis that attempts to combine structure and agency. Giddens (1984) offers an approach that integrates the two, seeing them as two sides of the same coin. He offers a theory of 'structuration' that attempts to take full account of both structure and agency. He also gives an account of structures rather different from any described hitherto. Social structures are composed of two elements: rules and resources. Rules are those elements of social life which guide social encounters, offer regulation of those encounters and may be more or less formalised (as laws or as mores). Resources have two elements: first allocative, second authoritative. Allocative resources are raw materials, which exist in a 'virtual' state until they are actually exploited by people. Thus land does not become a resource until, through human action, it is used in some way. Authoritative resource is the ability to dominate others and, to a greater or lesser degree, determine their actions. Authority is grounded in language and knowledge, through which we know and share the world. The exercise of authority is what makes it a resource; therefore authority too is 'virtual' and is not possessed until it is used. The use of authority, in a transformative capacity in relation to the resources to which it is applied, is a demonstration of power. Power is therefore the capacity to transform or 'make a difference' to structures. Thus structures are themselves produced and reproduced by human action, but, unless in some way being affected by action, they too are 'virtual'. It is the human action that makes real structures and maintains and changes them over time. Giddens describes this as 'instantiation'.

Giddens thus suggests that structures do not simply constrain human action, as many of the previous analyses have argued, but also, to some extent, enable it. Without structures, humans would have no spheres within which to act. This also offers an explanation of why some structures endure over time and others become redundant or obsolete. Chapter 11 makes use of Giddens' ideas to explore the transformative capacity of nursing care.

Feminist approaches

Feminist approaches, because of their range and diversity, pose some problems in a short exposition of this kind, particularly in relation to what is included and excluded. Not all strands of feminist thought are included here; to do so would be beyond the scope of this text.

On the whole, feminist approaches reject the posture of rationalism or of objective enquiry implicit in the foregoing social theories. Such rejection stems from the invisibility of women in the analyses offered, which has created disenchantment with 'malestream' (Abbott and Wallace 1990a) theories. They all, to some extent, revolve around the notion of patriarchy, or male power and its dominance in the social world. Rich (1977) has provided a useful definition:

> Patriarchy is... a familial-social, ideological, political system in which men – by force, direct pressure or through ritual, law and language, customs, etiquette, education, and the division of labour, determine what part women shall or shall not play, and in which the female is everywhere subsumed under the male. It does not necessarily imply that no woman has power, or that all women in a given culture may not have certain powers.
>
> (Rich 1977: 57)

Varied feminist approaches take different standpoints both in explaining men's power and in identifying the means to address power imbalances between men and women. As Chapters 3, 5, 6 and 7 make clear, power issues in nursing cannot be explored without examining the influence of patriarchy on nursing and nursing work. Patriarchy as a cultural system pervades the organisations in which nurses work (see Chapters 3 and 5), their relationships with the medical profession (Chapter 7), their relationships with each other (Chapters 4 and 5), their professional status (Chapter 2), their place in the labour market (Chapter 6) and the low status and invisibility of caring work.

Liberal feminism

Liberal feminists have adopted a rationalist position, seeing inequalities between men and women as deriving from women's unequal access to rights and choices. Liberal feminists argue that women should have equal rights to men but are frequently relegated to the status of second-class citizens because they do not have equal access to structures that would admit them to society on equal terms. In this analysis, education systems, for example, have favoured boys and therefore men. Until recently, men were educated to act in the public world, while girls' experience of education prepared them for the private world of the family, fulfilling the stereotyped roles of wife and mother.

The solution to this situation has been seen as more or less entirely located within existing social structures. Women should use those elements of the system that have inherent in them transformative power, particularly the legal system. Changes in legislation will, over time, lead to equality of opportunity, creating the proverbial 'level playing field' upon which women and men can compete on equal terms.

Marxist feminism

Marxist feminism accepts the Marxist view that the educational and legal systems are part of the superstructure, shaped by the power relationships of the economic base. Marxist mainstream theory is essentially blind to women, although Engels (1972) argued that it is capitalist forms of organisation that oppress women. From a Marxist standpoint, the failure of liberal approaches to produce rapid change can be explained by a failure to address the root cause of female oppression. The essentially exploitative nature of capitalism created a situation in which men occupied the public space of work and women the private sphere of home and family. Capitalist conditions of labour, including long hours and physical labour, largely excluded women from the public world of work, leaving women with the domestic and caring labour associated with home and family. This advantaged men in the accumulation of property and wealth, and in this way the family reflects wider society, men enjoying ownership of the available resources and women and children being dependent upon them in monogamous relationships. Monogamy also serves the interests of the bourgeoisie as it is the best form of organisation to protect male inheritance and their control over their wives and offspring. Thus women's productivity and reproductivity is oppressed in the interests of male productivity and reproductivity. Essentially, then, capitalist relationships are the cause of women's oppression. As Chapter 6 explains, dual labour market theory offered further opportunities to explore the way in which capitalism's labour markets contributed to women's inequalities in terms of labour power and economic resources.

Zaretsky (1976) agrees with the analysis that capitalism changed social relationships in relation to male domination of the public sphere and female subordination in the private sphere, but argues that it only had the effect of institutionalising already emerging forms of family organisation. Thus, in essence, capitalism is not the cause of female oppression but instead has been a major force in its perpetuation. Barrett (1980) points out that working-class men, as well as capitalists, benefit from women's labour and suggests that patriarchy and capitalism reinforce each other, thereby perpetuating male dominance. This approach, often described as 'dual systems theory', has been elaborated by Hartmann (1979, 1981), who has explored the way in which job segregation by sex and assumptions about the importance of a male wage being high enough to support a wife and children have facilitated male dominance both within the labour market and within the family. Trade unions served to secure gains for working men at the expense of working women, many of whom worked part time. Feminist analyses played an important role in uncovering patriarchal practices that sustained gender inequalities in paid work.

Radical feminism

Radical feminists argue that the oppression of women and children is the oldest and most extreme form of oppression in human relationships, pre-dating the emergence of capitalism as a form of social organisation. They argue that it is not class that is the significant element but gender itself.

Firestone (1972) contends that it is men's desire to control female biological capacity to reproduce, rather than their access to economic resources, that has led to women's oppressed status. Men's sexuality is seen as at the heart of male domination in that patriarchal culture is constructed to support male power over women through constructions that constrain women. Public and personal constructions of attractiveness, sexual power, appropriate dress, healthy bodies, dominance and submissiveness in sexual relationships and appropriate and inappropriate touch all affect personal and public relations between men and women.

In health and health care, radical feminists have identified the role that heterosexuality has played in the construction of 'normality' in medicalised views of women, and health service control over reproduction has been seen as deriving from and perpetuating male dominance (Stanworth 1987). Kelly (1988) has argued that our common sense definitions of what constitutes violence reflect men's ideas and do not reflect the range of male behaviours that women can perceive as threatening. Women's experience of male violence may be both hidden and pervasive, seriously affecting their well-being.

The solution offered by radical feminists is that of challenge and separation rather than reform and accommodation. Women have been encouraged to seize control of their own reproduction, to challenge the legality of pornography (Dworkin 1981, MacKinnon 1989) and to promote and protect their interests through collective action. The widespread establishment of hostels for battered women, rape crisis centres and telephone lines, and incest survivors and self-help groups attests to the success of such action and strategies. The importance of both sexuality and abuse in women's health makes an understanding of radical feminist approaches to male power particularly pertinent to nurses.

Feminist thought in the 1990s

Although liberal feminism, Marxist feminism and radical feminism developed in the 1970s as the main strands in feminist thought, later feminist writings have moved beyond these classifications, largely through a recognition that all these approaches failed to acknowledge the diversity of women's experiences. Feminist analyses appeared to focus on the interests of women who were white and heterosexual. The challenge to acknowledge diversity has been led by black feminists (Collins 1990) and lesbian authors, but it has many strands, including a concern with the way in which cultural and structural processes construct gender and sexualities, and hence identities. Post-structuralist or postmodern feminisms explore the processes by which subjectivity is shaped, expressed and fractured, offering possibilities that suggest a fluidity in sexual and gender identities and relationships, implying liberation of the self. Nevertheless, other feminist writers are also particularly interested in the body and the way in which it is 'inscribed within particular sets of power relations and can be read as a marker of difference (of gender, "race", class and sexuality)' (Stacey 1997: 70). There is much of interest for nurses among this literature, but to explore the subtleties of the strands of argument is beyond the scope of this book.

Other developments in feminist thought include what Porter (1998) has described as cultural feminism and standpoint feminism, positions that celebrate women's difference, presenting radically different views of morality and knowledge, views that can offer much to nurses in an exploration of the value and nature of knowledge about care. The recognition of the links between power and knowledge, however, is Foucault's contribution to our understanding of power.

Postmodern approaches

In essence, postmodern stances disagree with the theories considered up to now, all of which are grounded, to a greater or lesser extent, in a search for rational explanations. Postmodernists argue that there is no one way of examining a phenomenon, so there cannot be any single truth or reality, but that all things exist in a state of relativism. They argue that accepting and understanding difference offers an alternative theoretical position. It is not easy precisely to define postmodernism because of its central tenet of uncertainty. Lyotard (1984: xxiv) argues that the postmodern approach requires 'incredulity towards metanarratives', that is, that one should always be sceptical of any theory that claims an overarching and complete explanation of the social (or any other) world.

A central theme of Foucault's work is that of power. He argues (1980) that all knowledge is the product of power relations and that we need to understand how power produces knowledge. In his analysis, power and knowledge are closely related and do not exist in isolation from one another. Knowledge is constructed either to control nature or to influence the behaviour of others; therefore knowledge equals power. Significant to Foucault's analysis is 'discourse', commonly accepted assumptions that claim to explain reality and therefore form a base for knowledge. Discourses can exist simultaneously around any given phenomenon, some more dominant than others, some complementary and others not.

Foucault does not explain power in the same way as the theorists previously presented, although occasional similarities emerge. He is not unlike Giddens in that his explanation is not based in structures or institutions, which he sees as 'terminal forms' (1979: 92) derived from individual interactions. Instead, he sees power as evident at the point of interaction between individuals. Moreover, power is not held consistently by one or more social groups but emerges in and from their interactions. The demonstration of power lies in the unequal outcomes for the actors involved. However, because power is constantly present and widespread, it is produced and reproduced in all relationships, so any inequality of outcome is not necessarily a long-lived one, since the exercise of power always produces resistance as power and resistance are different sides of the same coin.

Power, in modern society, operates through a mechanism Foucault calls 'panopticism' (1991a [1975]), literally 'all-seeing', a form of constant surveillance to which we have become so accustomed that we apply it to ourselves, constantly monitoring our own behaviour and judging it against standards created by 'normalising judgment' (Merquior 1991: 94); thus we act as our own moral guardians in a process Foucault called 'subjectification' (Rabinow 1991). 'Normalising judgements' are produced by experts using their knowledge to define what is 'normal', and thus the 'abnormal' (the 'criminal', the 'insane', the 'sick') are drawn more tightly into the net of the experts and more evident forms of surveillance; for example, prisons, hospitals or special 'homes' for disabled people are created, ostensibly to assist them back to 'normality'. Chapter 8 adopts a Foucauldian analysis to explore the potential for teamworking in community care.

Foucault makes a specific case for medicine (1976) and the construction of the patient through a form of surveillance he called 'medical gaze'. In this analysis, the patient is reduced, through medical knowledge and all its artefacts, to nothing more than a biological machine that displays pathological behaviour, which may or may not be beyond repair. While this may be of instrumental value, it does have the effect of depersonalising the patient and denying his or her life experience. One need only think of the consequences of medicalising childbirth to be aware of the dangers of pathologising normal processes. Critiques of this sort have, however, resulted in a broadening of the sphere of interest of medicine and nursing to include the whole person, thus broadening the field of enquiry and (perhaps) subjectifying individuals, rather than simply objectifying them. This Foucault called 'pastoral power' (Porter 1998), which opens up even the most intimate areas of the patient's life to surveillance.

Such intimacy is intrinsic to nursing. Just as the physical nature of nursing care places a special responsibility on nurses to reflect on the difference between authority and coercion, so the potential for nursing surveillance places a special responsibility on nurses to recognise the power of health professionals to inscribe negative identities to those in their care. Part IV explores ways in which nurses can themselves resist disabling discourses and seek new modes of nursing practice grounded in a deeper understanding of the constraints and potential of what Fox (1993), writing from a postmodern standpoint, describes as 'care-as-gift'.

2 Power and professions

Geoff Wilkinson and Margaret Miers

Introduction

Nurses' ability or inability to work as autonomous professionals is central to any analysis of power and nursing. Nursing's status as work, as an occupation, as a profession or a semi-profession affects nurses' relationship to the state, their role in the health care team and their work with patients and clients. Whether and how well those who provide nursing care are paid, managed, educated, promoted and involved in decision making has often been identified as being dependent on the professional status, or lack of it, of nursing. This is not surprising. Occupations regarded as professions earn more and enjoy more control and higher social status than do many non-professional jobs. Professions are seen as having a special place within society.

Functionalism and professions

Functionalist sociologists have explained the importance of professions by noting the contributions they make to the well-being of society. The knowledge and skills that allow professionals to serve the needs of society are acquired over a lengthy period of education and training through which they are socialised into an ethic of service. In return for the altruism deemed implicit in the willingness to study for professional qualifications and for the commitment to placing service to the community before self- interest, professionals are rewarded by high earnings and prestige. Functionalist explanations were developed in the 1950s and 60s (Greenwood 1957, Carr-Saunders and Wilson 1962, Barber 1963). A linked approach, the trait approach, is exemplified by Greenwood's five distinctive characteristics of a profession: (1) a basis of systematic theory, (2) authority recognised by the clientele, (3) community sanction of this authority,

(4) a code of ethics, and (5) a professional culture sustained by professional associations. Similarly, Barber identified four 'essential attributes' of a profession that explained both its importance to society and the rewards it gained. These attributes were (1) possession of a body of systematic and generalised knowledge, (2) motivation for public service rather than personal gain, (3) behaviour controlled by a code of ethics, regulated by a professional association and learned through prolonged education and training, and (4) prestige and financial rewards accorded in recognition of achievement. Identifying the core characteristics of a profession, despite the fact that agreement about specific traits was elusive, allowed sociologists to identify occupations that did not warrant full professional status. Nursing, like social work, was defined as a semi-profession because it lacked a systematic knowledge base, was based on skills rather than knowledge and lacked independent self-government in the workplace (Etzioni 1969). Nursing's dependence on medical knowledge and on medical control over the organisation of nursing work meant that nurses lacked autonomy and that their level of rewards, authority and community sanction of that authority remained subordinate to doctors.

Nurses using a trait approach to the analysis of the professions could deduce that it was a lack of systematic knowledge and practice based on skills, rather than nursing theory, that prevented nursing from achieving full professional status. The solution could be seen as the development of nursing theory and approaches to the assessment and delivery of patient care that would clearly differentiate nursing from medicine. The development of independent nursing theories, models and the hegemonic nursing process accompanied the development of a hierarchy of nursing management after the Salmon Report in 1968 and coincided with the unification of nursing's professional bodies under the umbrella of the United Kingdom Central Council for Nursing, Midwifery and Health Visiting (UKCC). All these factors could be seen to contribute to giving nurses increased control over nursing and to gaining increased authority and community sanction through an independent knowledge base.

This is not the book in which to explore the inherent strengths and limitations of nursing theories and nursing models or the importance to nursing of implementing a planned approach to care through the nursing process. As Jolley (1989) noted, 'protagonists of the Nursing Process approach to care see it as instrumental in making the distinction between nursing and medicine clear' (p. 15). Further developments of what came to be described (albeit briefly) as the 'new nursing' (Salvage 1992), an approach based on the deliberate delineation of nursing and medicine, included primary nursing, a system of organising nursing care that emphasised the autonomy of nursing and its separation from medicine. (Chapter 5 offers some reflections on the limitations of this approach.) In Savage's research study, discussed in Chapter 5, primary nursing could be seen as creating barriers between medicine and nursing, and could not be sustained during health service cuts (Savage 1995). Nursing theories can be criticised for their inability to provide a systematic knowledge base from which to derive general principles for nursing care. In many areas of practice, general principles of care remained dependent on knowledge shared with, if not owned by, doctors and other professionals in the care team. Miller (1989) found that, whereas nursing theories provided useful maps for the inexperienced and were essential teaching guides, for the experienced nurse their use in practice was of limited value. This is a curious position for a developing profession to find itself in. The knowledge base it claims as its own is useful for the beginner but fails the proficient and thus must fail to provide an adequate basis for the development of nursing practice and nursing as a profession.

Critiques of functionalist and trait approaches

If the development of nursing theories and models was part of a professionalising strategy for the empowerment of nurses, a strategy based on attempts to ensure that nursing could claim the 'traits' of a profession, its inadequacy as a strategy for increasing nursing's autonomy and influence can be seen as deriving in part from the naïvety of functionalism as an analysis of health care or professionalism. Functionalism's limitations as an approach to understanding professional prestige are many. Far from being an explanation of professional power, functionalist and trait approaches were criticised for being a justification of the privileged position of specific occupational groups such as doctors and lawyers at a particular historical time. The assumptions that professions make important contributions to society, that they serve the interests of all rather than of particular groups and that they are motivated by altruism rather than self-interest have all been questioned.

Freidson saw a profession as an occupation that has succeeded in controlling its own work and has been granted legitimate autonomy, usually through the state. Freidson (1970) acknowledged the possibility that the professional 'may, in conforming to the norms of his profession, perform at the same time a disservice to the public whose interests the profession supposedly supports and satisfies'. Johnson (1972) saw professions not as neutral occupational groups but as institutionalised means of controlling occupational activities, particularly those involving relationships between a producer and consumer. He identified three different types of control within professional organisations: collegiate, in which power is exercised by members; patronage, in which power is negotiated between professionals and those who pay directly for their services; and state mediation, in which the state mediates between the profession and the service users. Both Freidson's and Johnson's analyses draw out the power relationships involved in professional activity. Professionals have the autonomy, granted through the state, to serve each other's interests rather than those of the public; professional power is dependent on the state, which can intervene in professional activity through managerial, financial and bureaucratic control; service users may control professional activity either through directly purchasing services or through the mediation of the state. In such analyses of professions, power becomes central and the service ideal is lost. Understandably, therefore, some authors have raised questions about the desirability of professional status for nursing (Salvage 1985, Jolley 1989, Davies 1995).

Professionalisation and social closure

Porter (1998) has noted Johnson's dependency on the ideas of Max Weber (1968), particularly the importance of market mechanisms in determining the status and rewards of particular occupations. Johnson (1972) identified professions' strategies of occupational control as resting on the restriction of entry to the profession, thereby ensuring low supply and high demand, the maintenance of occupational homogeneity, sustained through 'the myth of equal competence' (Porter 1998: 66) and favourable image-building. Porter links Weber's recognition of the importance of social closure and monopolisation as market mechanisms to Parkin's further elaboration of processes of social closure, notably social closure as exclusion and social closure as usurpation (Parkin 1979). Social closure by exclusion occurs through restricting access to resources and opportunities such as education and training, and social closure by usurpation occurs through groups challenging the restrictive practices and privileges of an advantaged minority in order to gain advantage for themselves. Viewed in this way, it is obvious that the process of gaining, retaining and restricting professional skills, knowledge and roles is a highly contested one.

Witz (1992) has argued that nursing and midwifery have adopted dual closure strategies in the pursuit of occupational control, thereby seeking more secure professional autonomy and status. As Porter's summary makes clear, Witz identified the campaign for nursing registration as a dual closure strategy in which a centralised system of control through state registration was sought, with a demand that nurses should have the right to govern themselves. A third demand was a uniportal system of entry, which would have allowed for centralised control over education and training. These demands could be seen as an attempt at both exclusion and usurpation, since their success could have reduced the freedom of the voluntary hospital authorities and challenged medicine's control over the organisation of nurses' work. Although registration was granted in 1919 and a centralised body, the General Nursing Council, was established, the Council did not achieve autonomy over education, training, pay and conditions, and the routes into nursing remained diverse. Nevertheless, it can be argued that nursing continued to pursue dual closure strategies in order to improve its market position and professional power. The UKCC, established in 1979, has a majority of elected members and has the power to establish and police professional rules, and control registration. The Project 2000 educational reforms (UKCC 1986) established one entry gate through abolishing the 2-year enrolled nurse educational programme and denying unqualified staff the title of 'nurse'.

Auxiliary nurses have largely been replaced by health care assistants. Porter (1995a) has also argued that the development of the nursing process is a dual closure strategy, challenging medical monopoly but also furthering the exclusion of nurses without registered status by restricting care planning and assessment to first-level nurses. As a strategy for professional empowerment, however, Porter found the nursing process singularly ineffective. Care plans were not used as 'aids to care' (Porter 1998: 79) although they were used as records of work done (with the potential to stand as legal documents). Furthermore, the care plans remained framed within a medical assessment of needs and treatment. While this is perhaps unsurprising, given the intensive care setting in which Porter completed his field work, it nevertheless reinforces doubts about the ability of nursing theories and the nursing process to develop nursing expertise and enhance the professional status of nursing.

Marxist critiques of professional power

Yet again, however, the limitations in the closure strategy may not lie in the nursing process but in the Weberian (in addition to the functionalist/trait) approach to the analysis of professions. Two further theoretical approaches must be explored, namely Marxism and feminisms. As Porter (1998: 81) makes clear:

> Marxists criticise the Weberian focus on market arrangements on the grounds that it is unable to explain why those market arrangements take the form that they do... Marxists argue that we need to look at the material conditions that pertain... The distinctiveness of capitalist societies lies in the form of exploitation they entail, which is embedded in the relations of production between the owners and non-owners of the means of production.

In Marx's analysis of stratification, skill ownership may be seen as irrelevant except in so far as the skills are part of the relationships of production and are used in support of the interests of the owners of the means of production. Professional skills can be so used, through maintaining the health and welfare of the workforce at minimal cost. Non-professional skills are cheap, and keeping the costs of skills low benefits those with the purchasing capital. From this analysis, it is the reciprocal legitimising role of the professions and the state, and the circumstances in which this takes place that are of interest. However, from the point of view of a state-funded health service, a rise in professional status for half of its workforce (nurses) would be expensive and hence unlikely to be encouraged. Opportunities for the movement of a semi-profession to full professional status and rewards would be minimised by the increased labour costs, unless closure by usurpation could reduce the costs of a more expensive professional commodity (doctors) and thus fund the raised salary costs that may derive from the nursing profession's successful closure by exclusion. Chapter 6 explores the place of nurses in the labour market.

Illich (1977) regarded the medical profession as a threat to health. He saw the disabling impact of professional control as an epidemic, an epidemic of iatrogenesis, that is, of physician origin. Illich (1977: 16) argued:

> A professional and physician-based health-care system that has grown beyond critical bounds is sickening for three reasons: it must produce clinical damage that outweighs its potential benefits; it cannot but enhance even as it obscures the political conditions that render society unhealthy; and it tends to mystify and to expropriate the power of the individual to heal himself and to shape his or her environment.

Thus, within a capitalist society, a physician-based health care system could be seen as contributing to ill health, obscuring yet enhancing the class-based inequalities and relationships (political conditions) that produce ill health and disempowering individuals by professional expropriation of the power to heal. Such an analysis of health care presents the medical profession as all powerful yet disabling. As part of the health care system, nurses could appear as less powerful yet still disabling. This is an analysis of professional power that contrasts sharply with any assumptions about a professional ethic of care and consequently seems to offer nothing to nursing. Illich's identification of limits to medicine can be seen as fostering a growth in complementary and alternative approaches to healing, approaches that some nurses have deliberately included in their practice (Coward 1990).

A Marxist critique of professionalism can also illuminate the inequalities inherent in the processes of professional recruitment and advancement. As Hugman (1991) notes, 'the UK pattern of racism in health and welfare employment is an institutional expression of the white racism which finds its origins in Western Europe' and in colonialism (p. 146). In nursing, status as enrolled or registered nurses helped discriminatory practices to create a primary and secondary labour market in which white nurses dominated nursing hierarchies while black nurses, recruited during post-Second World War labour shortages, were denied opportunities for career progression (Doyal *et al.* 1981). As Chapter 4 indicates, class also played its part in the development of nursing élites. This lack of equality of opportunity within the profession, explored by Jones (1994), was mirrored by discriminatory practices towards clients. Chapters 9 and 12 both explore the possibilities of reducing the disabling power of professional practice as it affects particular client groups: the elderly, and lesbians and gay men. Such discrimination can be seen in part as a consequence of the cultural consequences (cultural iatrogenesis) of medical power, as presented by Illich and other critics of medicalisation (Zola 1975).

Patriarchy and professions: gender analyses

Feminist writers have argued that professions are patriarchal structures that inherently discriminate against women. The gendered nature of the organisation of health work is discussed in Chapters 3 and 5. The influence of gender on the relationship between nurses and doctors is also explored in Chapter 7. Witz (1992) links the analysis of professionalising strategies of closure to the analysis of gender, arguing that 'the agents of closure practices are gendered so gender may form the basis of solidarity between men and women' (p. 51). However, Witz notes that the emphasis on professionalising projects as process neglects the importance of structure: 'Power is a built-in attribute of closure, so there is a one-sided emphasis on the exercise of power and a neglect of the mere possession of power' (p. 51). The structures Witz is interested in are patriarchal structures in which men hold power. Professions are such structures. Witz argues that all professionalising strategies are necessarily gendered by the gender of the strategists and hence refers to 'gendered strategies and patriarchal structures', thereby establishing that:

> gendered actors who are engaged in professional projects as strategic courses of action will have differential access to the tactical means of achieving their aims in a patriarchal society within which male power is institutionalised and organised. (p. 52)

Whereas this is easily illustrated through the history of nursing, given that access to universities, the means of credentialism for the dominant professions, medicine and the law, was denied to women, the extent to which nursing is currently subjected to the power of patriarchal structures is less obvious. Nevertheless, as the following chapters illustrate, the gendered nature of structures can be noted in the invisibility of nurses' work and the subtleties of factors such as posture and use of space. Chapter 5 implies that assumptions about professional interactional styles can be gendered.

Celia Davies has extended the analysis of the links between professions and patriarchy. She argues that the notion of profession celebrates a masculine vision of expertise. 'Professional knowledge is gained by dint of a lengthy and heroic individual effort. This effort is a project involving mastery, resulting in knowledge as a "possession" of the autonomous individual' (Davies 1995: 59). This masculine model of professionalism can be seen as inappropriate for nursing, which relies on interpersonal co-operation between nurses and clients and nurses and other professionals rather than autonomous mastery. Davies notes that criticisms of the monopolistic inward-looking tendencies of professionalism derive from questions about costs, about the effectiveness of professional interventions and about professionals' ability or inability to work co-operatively to meet users' needs. Chapter 8 explores the issue of multiprofessional teamwork from a Foucauldian perspective, noting the difficulties that individual professions have in recognising the extent to which specific professional discourses frame approaches to assessment and service delivery. Government impatience with the disabling power of professions led, during the 1980s and early 1990s, to the privatisation and deregulation of public services, thus reducing the mediating beneficence of the state as the upholder of professional power. However, paradoxically, it also led to an increase in systems of governmentality (Foucault 1991), that is, subtle and systematic systems of formal control, through, for example, *Health of the Nation* (DoH 1992a) targets and the surveillance necessary to promote health.

Davies develops Stacey's view that the old model of professionalism is outdated (Stacey 1992) and outlines a model of 'new professionalism', drawing on the ideas of Hugman (1991), who advocates increased professional–client partnership and participation, and Schön (1983), who sees reflective practice rather than scientific knowledge as a source of professional expertise. Davies' 'new professionalism', outlined in Chapter 14, involves 'dislodging the gendered model of profession' and acknowledging the importance of the engaged and interdependent nature of professional practice in which an 'embodied use of self' is part of the 'therapeutic encounter' and the professional is a 'creator of an active community in which a solution can be negotiated' and a 'reflective user of experience and expertise' (Davies 1995: 149–150). The gendered thought that lies behind a masculine model of professional power trivialises and fails to acknowledge the work traditionally done by women. Davies' 'new professionalism' revalues communicative, engaged, embodied negotiation and support. This is a caring practitioner model of nursing practice.

Although Davies' model of new professionalism emerges through a feminist critique of professional power, it is a model which concurs with many analyses of the need to change professional practice to foster user empowerment. The examples of professional practice explored in this book demonstrate the influence of communicative, engaged care. Perhaps this is unsurprising. Functionalism suggests that professionals gain status in the community because of the importance of the service they perform and their denial of self-interest. It is assumed that their ability to perform the service rests on specialised knowledge acquired through a prolonged education and training that is under the direction of the professional body. Apparently lacking its own specialised knowledge base, nursing has developed its own theories, models and approaches, and consolidated the educational experience of its neophytes through the development of higher education qualifications. Nursing has thus pursued a professionalising project. Paradoxically, some of nursing's academic development may have been resting on a distorted understanding of the nature of the service nurses provide, the skills they use and the origin of community admiration and support for nurses. Davies claims that nurses 'face issues of reconciling professionalism and caring as dilemmas of daily practice' (Davies 1995: 145). Yet the specific and functionally important service that nurses provide and which brings them the privileged status of a profession may be the provision of care and support to vulnerable strangers. If so, gendered strategists (in Witz's terms) working within patriarchal structures may themselves have denigrated the 'power' of nurses' contribution – the contribution of care – to individuals and the community. Seeking the development of a formalised knowledge base without ensuring that it relates adequately to the practice of interpersonal care and support can appear to deny the importance of practice. Closure strategies that are founded on the rhetoric, rather than the analysis, of expertise are likely to fail irrespective of the policy, political and patriarchal or matriarchal context.

Conclusion

It seems appropriate, in a text in a *Sociology and Nursing Practice* series, to identify the problematic relationship between nursing knowledge and nursing skills as possibly a key yet neglected element in the success of nursing's professionalising strategies. The trait approach's emphasis on a systematic body of knowledge appears to take for granted the fact that the theory base will underpin, support and develop skills. Nursing theories and nursing models, however, have failed to emphasise the environmental or social context of health and social care, and may thereby minimise the use of theoretical knowledge in practice. Practice always takes place in a social context. Sociological knowledge, however, may equally fail to illuminate practice. Whereas an educational emphasis on *nursing* as opposed to biological and psychological as well as sociological knowledge may inhibit the successful application of knowledge to the assessment and care of clients in varied health statuses and health care settings, so too might an educational emphasis on specialist knowledge as opposed to nursing. In some settings, knowledge about anatomy and physiology may be crucial to a nurse's ability to intervene effectively. In others, knowledge about biological sciences may have limited application. As May has pointed out, a limited understanding of the *complexity* of using a biopsychosocial approach to nursing care can turn nurses' willingness and wish to empower clients into surveillance through the therapeutic gaze (May 1992a).

Many of the following chapters attempt to identify aspects of the social context (gendered assumptions, élitism, hierarchies, labour costs, medical power, professional discourses, hetero-sexism, ageism, community ignorance and prejudice about learning disabilities and mental illness) that both disempower nurses and inhibit their ability to empower clients. The chapters also identify the interpersonal, negotiating, teamwork and supportive skills that, together with changing the environment of care, may alter power balances within the health care team in its broadest sense, that is, including carers and clients. The assumptions are that nurses can and do 'make a difference', but the empowerment that clients may derive from the embodied nature of nurses' care has yet to be explored in an explicit and accessible manner that acknowledges the physicality and identity of both client and nurse. If skills of empowerment remain cognitively hidden, beyond analysis and therefore invisible, the development of relevant knowledge is at best haphazard.

Even a clear relationship between knowledge and skills would not now necessarily enhance nursing's professional status. The current policy and professional emphasis on user involvement (see Chapters 9 and 10) in health and social care recognises that professionals' position in society has rested on their ability to serve (or appear to serve) the interests of society. The outcomes of professional activity must be valued by their clients. Nurses' strength is their popularity, a popularity that may well rest in their embodiment of the service ethic which can be seen as at the heart of professionalism. As Hugman notes:

> the 'service ethic' as an ideal points to the desirability of developing more open relationships between professionals and service users to make an ethic of professional service possible. In this sense the ethics of a profession are not abstract moral values, but are related to the social relationships within which professionals act... these are relationships of power.
> (1991: 224)

Hugman's aim is our aim:

> to recognise explicitly the aspects of power in caring professions, and from the questions which are raised by the consideration of power to

> seek the development of caring professions which increasingly are directed towards empowering their members and those who use their services. (p. 224)

Lupton (1996) has noted the rationalist nature of the consumerist movement, which supports the involvement of users in service provision. Lupton sees the consumerist movement as arguably:

> an attempt to deal with uncertainty and anxiety by evoking rationalist anti authoritarianism against an 'other'... defined as controlling.
>
> (1996: 169)

Those in control are professionals, yet Lupton reminds us that trust minimises the danger of risk (Giddens 1990) and remains an element in professional–client relationships in health care settings, especially when individuals are seriously ill or disabled. Lupton argues that:

> while the consumerist approach tends to represent people as autonomous individuals who are self reliant, we need to acknowledge the emotional ties that bind people to each other in ways of which they are not often fully aware. There are times in which people derive reassurance and comfort from allowing themselves to become dependent upon others: the experience of acute pain or serious illness is often one of these times. (p. 169)

Fox (1993) has noted the reciprocal nature of staff–patient trust:

> Patients trust staff not to hurt them unduly, to treat them with compassion and as fellow humans, not to exploit them for sexual fantasy or actual use, not to breach confidentiality. Staff trust patients to co-operate and submit to the technologies and competencies claimed by the discipline.
>
> (1993: 42)

Fox's contract is the contract between professions and society played out in individual caring contact. Relationships of power are relationships of trust or distrust.

In considering the empowering potential of professional status for both nurses and their clients, this chapter has noted the importance of developing a more sensitive analysis of the embodied nature of nursing skills as well as the structures within which nursing is practised. This analysis begins in the following chapters.

PART II

Nurses' relationships with nurses

3 Power, gender and nursing work

Gill Mowforth

Introduction

The concepts of gender and power and their manifestation at the macro and micro levels within nursing are examined in this chapter. In the past, gender has often been excluded from theoretical analyses of power. The reason for this may be that most of the writers were male. Feminist approaches have forced gender issues to become more visible within the literature. The impact of feminism on our thinking on gender and on our behaviour cannot be minimised. However, while many areas of women's lives have been explored in the literature (Oakley 1972, Phillips 1987, Barrett and McIntosh 1991, Tong 1992, Graham 1993, Charles and Hughes-Freeland 1996), few writers have turned their attention to nurses' work as paid carers in the same detail. Walby *et al.* (1994), however, undertook a detailed study into medicine and nursing, which involved exploring power issues and nursing work.

Gender

Gender is a descriptive concept that is useful for uncovering differences between male and female experiences, behaviour and position within society. Gender can also shape an individual's opportunity for education, work, reproduction, authority and the chance to make a contribution to a culture or to the production of its knowledge (Lorber 1991). In other words, there is no part of our lives in which gender issues are not relevant. However, differences in opportunities do not explain why the relations between men and women frequently seem to involve domination and subordination. Gender has a bearing on how we relate to each other, first as boys and girls, then as men and women. Gender affects us when we attend or work within institutions or in the private sphere (Hugman 1991). Social life is deeply gendered, and it is often at the level of social relations that one can detect the fault line between boys and girls, men and women. Walby *et al.* (1994) see studies on gender as being divided between studies at the attribution level, which encompasses psychosocial explanations (why we are who or what we are) (Gilligan 1982), and the structural and organisational level as described by Witz and Savage (1992), and Davies (1992). Much of the recent literature has focused on the latter.

In relation to medicine and nursing, Walby *et al.* (1994) have asserted that gender is relevant when looking at the internal hierarchy of each profession. They emphasised that gender is an indispensable concept when examining the structures in which nurses find themselves. Celia Davies has argued that gender is not imported into institutions and workplaces but is embedded in their structures. This, she comments, will not be eradicated by the 'equal opportunities police' (Davies 1992: 230). Nursing is a good starting place for observing how gender relations are manifested, not only between men and women, but also between women and between men. One of the major criticisms of gender attribution theory over the past few years has been that masculinity and femininity are not consistent attributes that all men and all women possess; they are not separate and complementary but must be understood in relation to each other (Davies 1992). However, masculinity and femininity often act as cultural codes, and this is reflected in many organisations that are not gender neutral. What is expected of a man and what assumptions can be made of a woman are often relived in what Acker (1991) has described as organisational logic. These writers have moved beyond simplistic feminist analyses. They acknowledge that masculinity and femininity are powerful images and have been used to great effect in promoting nursing as a nurturing and caring profession. One of the problems of gender theory is that power imbalances tend to be reflected in other inequalities as well. In other words, gender inequalities often become conflated with those of class, race, age or disability. There is often not one single source. Hence a feminist search for universal explanations is now misplaced. Nurses are expected to care in a masculinist world, which both men and women find difficult. Indeed, Connell (1987) has argued that the main axis of the power structure of gender relations is the connection of authority with masculinity. This link shapes the experience of both men and women.

Feminist approaches to analysing gender

Gender became a central theme for many feminist writers during the 1960s and 70s. Feminist writers at that time ignored the diversity of women's experience associated with class, race, age and disability. Unbalanced relationships were viewed as the inevitable result of patriarchal structures of domination. This lack of attention to diversity has never been satisfactorily explained other than to suggest that those issues were not considered essential to many of the women who were prominent in the women's movement during that time. Phillips (1987) has argued that it has been an easy criticism to level at the women who led the movement, representing women as though they were all heterosexual, white and middle class. Male oppression was the challenge to the feminist movement at the time. Within the social context of those years, women and men were often described as a homogeneous group, a unitary category. Men as a category were seen as symbols of the patriarchy. Patriarchy was defined as the legitimate authority given to men solely on the grounds of their gender. Patriarchal domination could be observed in the private and public domain, that is, in the home and the workplace. In subsequent decades, feminists developed new knowledge about women's lives that challenged that universality. Literature began to reflect differences between women and their situation (Collins 1990). The politics of diversity became more apparent; it demanded a voice and a platform where the contradictions became obvious. It was a confusing time as the unified category known as 'woman' was challenged (Razmanoglu 1989).

Just as the concept of universality of women has now become problematic for feminists, so has the other key concept known as 'patriarchy'. Walby (1990) suggested that patriarchy could be analysed in terms of six main areas of our lives: paid work, domestic work, the state, male violence, sexuality and culture. She argued that patriarchy is mediated through ideology, which enables men to gain dominance over women, within those structures. Other authors saw patriarchy rooted in the subordination of women by men in contemporary industrial societies as having an economic base (Hartmann 1976). Hartmann described patriarchy thus: 'A set of social relations which has a material base and in which there are hierarchical relations between men and a solidarity among them which enables them to control women. Patriarchy is thus the system of male oppression of women' (cited in Carter 1994: 368). If we do accept that patriarchy is universal, in the sense that all men have power over all women, that would make all women victims of oppression, an untenable generalisation. Within patriarchal societies, women also have power over other women. Too many generalisations about male domination can lead us to deny the contradictions in womens' lives.

Gender and power

The issue of power has been treated differently by various feminist approaches. Liberal feminists see power as being diffused throughout society and would use legislation to equalise any power imbalances. Marxist feminists identify power as being part of organisational structures and gender relationships that intersect with the particular mode of production of the time. This is both within the home and in the public arena. Radical feminists locate male power within most social structures and argue that it is supported in the main by an ideology that upholds the biological basis of male strength through socialisation, culture and social structures, which give men a dominant position (Millett 1970). They would look for alternative modes of production that are not dependent on patriarchal power as they would define it (Razmanoglu 1989).

Feminist theories have uncovered the central concept of gender and have facilitated studies in every realm of womens' lives. Davis (1991) writes that if we wished to explore power issues in a more detailed way using a feminist perspective, it would be possible to use two approaches. First, gender can be taken as the central concept, and an attempt can then be made to develop a feminist theory on gender and power. This approach assumes that power between the sexes can best be understood in terms of gender relations. The second approach would take power as the central concept, and gender relations would be only part of the analysis. In other words, the feminist explanations would be part of the analysis but would not exclude other theories or approaches. There cannot be one general feminist theory on power because it would be too limiting if it were based only on gender relations. However, it is important that gender relations are identified. If not, they may be ignored altogether.

Many writers have either chosen to ignore or are blind to gender issues when writing on power. Many of the theories on power are grand in design and are embedded in organisational and structural explanation. For Giddens (1984), power is one of several important concepts at which the intersection of structures and human agency are brought together. He would see power as an enabling force, even though it can be a constraining one, involving relations of dependency and autonomy. This, he would argue, is absolutely intrinsic to human actions and social interactions. Giddens described power as Janus-faced, unlike Lukes' (1974) three dimensions of power or Gramsci's (1916) ideological hegemonic power. Foucault (1980), like Giddens, saw power as a productive and positive force rather than merely a negative and repressive one. However, he excluded women from his analyses and theories. He explored power only as it is located in institutions and not from the individual subject's perspective. One of his main arguments was that, wherever power was uncovered, so too was resistance. Resistance was often to be found within the most rigid and intensely authoritarian regimes. However, he did not necessarily see resistance as the use of force; instead it was through the manipulation of power that resistance was at its most productive. Foucault did not perceive power as a static force either, residing in one person, but described it as a dynamic entity, which was not dependent on legitimate authority within an organisation (MacNay 1994). The ideology of masculinity and authority is an important issue for nurses, as the ideological world can sometimes censor that which does not fit in. In the world of nursing work, it does this successfully by marginalising that which it wishes to exclude, causing nursing work to become invisible. Invisibility is something that will be returned to later in the chapter.

Gender, organisations and power

Davies and Rosser (1986) explored the possibility of discriminatory practices within the NHS and identified different career pathways that care workers were encouraged to take. This often proved to be excluding for the majority of women. These pathways Davies and Rosser described as hierarchy A and hierarchy B. Hierarchy A, or the 'golden pathway', contained most of the men and few of the women, while hierarchy B contained most of the women and few of the men and offered fewer career opportunities. The golden pathway attracted younger men, usually under 30 years of age, who were mobile and were able to travel at a moment's notice. Hierarchy B staff underpinned the 'golden pathway' because they had been in post for a long time and were able to offer a wealth of experience. The gap between the two hierarchies was very wide, and very limited movement took place between the two groups of staff. The work performed by hierarchy B staff was generally underrated by those on the hierarchy A pathway and was often invisible. Davies and Rosser felt that the climate was hostile to women because it compounded the historical evolution of a gendered labour process within health care work. This is mostly based on men's assumptions concerning women's abilities and preferences, thereby disadvantaging women. This is a good example of exclusion and marginalisation. Hence we can see that gender attribution theory was produced and reproduced within one section of the labour market. Male assumptions concerning women's career choices were echoed by female nurses. Davies and Rosser confronted female nurses with the fact that a disproportionate number of men were in positions of authority, even though women formed the majority of the workforce. The women often became quite hostile towards the interviewer and were adamant that they were at the level they had chosen to be. Davies and Rosser reached the conclusion that, while the NHS was not an overtly discriminatory employer, the cultural context in which workers found themselves had such a masculine agenda that other attributes had been marginalised.

The realisation that social structures are gendered has slowly evolved in feminist discourse (Acker 1991, Davies 1995). There is also a common sense, taken-for-granted, approach about organisations, which Acker describes as organisational logic. This, she states, is an indivisible part of all institutions. It is manifested in a number of ways, which all interact with each other. This then makes it difficult to challenge an organisation's gendered approach.

This has much relevance for nursing. Taking Acker's thesis, Davies (1995) has further explored nursing's organisational logic. Nursing has an observable division of labour in which men and women perform different jobs or men are in higher positions over women. Nearly 90 per cent of nursing's workforce is female, yet male nurses hold more of the top jobs (Jones 1994). Patterns of domination and subordination are frequently repeated in organisations, and Acker gives an example of how this can occur at meetings, with women taking their turn to speak and not interrupting the men. In nursing, this can be observed very clearly on some hospital ward rounds with a dominant consultant. Organisational logic also takes on a material form in respect of written rules and how certain jobs become evaluated. Within this logic, hierarchies get taken for granted and every job has a place within those hierarchies. Acker calls this an essential part of organisational logic. We can perhaps now understand how Davies and Rosser's interviewees were quite clear that it was their choice that they were where they were in the organisation. There is also an assumption that there are inextricable links between hierarchical positions and job complexity as defined by the organisation. The hierarchical divisions within an institution can also resonate with differences in power within the same occupational group, which is reflected in Catherine Hakim's (1979) work on vertical and horizontal segregation. Horizontal segregation occurs when men and women are working in different types of work, and vertical segregation refers to the concentration of men in higher grades within the same occupation. While horizontal segregation within nursing is not gender segregated, it appears so when vertical segregation is examined. It is a curious paradox that, while nursing makes up 90 per cent of the workforce within the NHS, and most of them are women, nurses are still marginalised (Beardshaw and Robinson 1990).

Nursing work and invisibility

Within nursing, the caring role has often become subordinated and interwoven with gendered assumptions about female attributes, about 'womanhood'. Oakley calls the link between nursing and womanhood the 'iron link' (Oakley 1984). Gamarnikow (1978) described the early relationship between doctor and nurse as being similar to that between father and mother, with the patient as the child. The nurse concentrated on the emotional environment of the patient while the doctor concentrated on the curing aspect of the role. In 1984, Oakley urged nurses to lift their veil to make themselves more visible; however, the invisibility of nurses' work has not been significantly changed despite an increase in men's influence within nursing. It certainly seems to be the case that nursing work has often been overlooked, excluded and marginalised within the health care arena. In adult nursing, the care of the person's body has been poorly understood by both the general public and managers. Perhaps it is because it has been closely associated with traditional care undertaken by women that it is taken for granted.

Many authors have written about the burden of care on carers (Finch and Groves 1983, Graham 1984, 1993, Dalley 1988), and they have painted a picture of the grinding physicality of caring for an ill or a disabled person, which may be quite invisible to the casual onlooker. For nurses, invisibility also constitutes a large part of their daily work. The effect of physicality on nurses' back problems, for example, has been largely invisible until recently; general concern by nurses, health and safety officers and lawyers has made the invisible visible, and improvements are now taking place, partly because of legislation. This has meant an investment in both equipment and training within the risk assessment arena.

During any healing process, emotional labour is often expended by the nurse, which is sometimes difficult to identify or evaluate. The term 'emotional labour' was originally used by Hochschild (1983) in her study of airline stewardesses and has since been used by authors analysing and commenting on nursing work (Smith 1988, James 1989). Hochschild identified various facets of emotional labour in which the stewardesses had direct contact with the public and tried to absorb and contain the passengers' feelings. The stewardesses were also encouraged by the management to regulate their own feelings and disguise them for the public's benefit. Hochschild noted a disparity between the stewardesses' feelings and how those feelings were being shown, this being achieved through training and socialisation. This is a significant piece of work for nurses as the control of their feelings, actions and reactions when confronted by patients' or clients' histories is important. Since the nursing process was implemented and individualised care for patients is now emphasised, the nurse is much more involved with the client group on the psychological as well as the physical level. These affective relationships become part of a nurse's emotional labour but are not always acknowledged. Time spent listening to patients and clients is often an invaluable aspect of the healing process but, again, can be invisible. The energy needed to manage or suppress feelings as a nurse is quite considerable, and adult nursing circles have probably been slower than other branches in realising how important supervision actually is for their work. The importance of listening can be illustrated by observing the nurse as listener in the accident and emergency department. Many nurses in that field may not appreciate how important it is to listen, for example, to a woman who has been the subject of male violence by a known man, or may minimise the importance of their role with the patient who self-harms and becomes a regular attender at their casualty department. It can be argued that the invisibility of some aspects of nursing work is a gender issue.

The evidence-based practice movement may contribute further to the invisibility of nursing work. Nursing outcomes are not easy to demonstrate through empirical methods. The complexity, the amount and the diversity of nursing work may become devalued. Walby *et al.* (1994) argued that, unless the nurses' body of professional knowledge helped in their patients' recovery, or contributed in any way to promoting their health, it would not be respected. A difficulty is that it is not always clear what a nurse's body of knowledge is. It may be invisible outside the nurse–patient relationship because the work is often conducted on an intimate level. It may be invisible because the work is frequently performed by women whose skills and expertise have been devalued by others who suggest that those attributes are innate and natural. The invisibility of parts of nursing work is frequently invisible to nurses themselves. They take for granted the loose parameters of the boundaries of their work, in the best interests of the patients. Through training and socialisation, individual nurses may remain unaware of how external interests shape their own desire to care and their ability to do so. Lukes' (1974) description of the third dimension of power can be revealed in nursing. Nurses would deny that they are exercising power over patients and would reject the idea they actually hold any power.

Similarly, they would deny that their own behaviour is possibly shaped by a patriarchal third face of power. Dowling and Barrett's (1991) work studying a group of pre-registration house officers in their first year discovered aspects of the house officers' work that were invisible to their consultants and senior doctors. Symptom control, diagnoses and communication with patients and relatives were the issues that were identified. An interesting outcome of the research was the amount of time identified during which senior nurses supervised the work of house officers. One research respondent stated that such supervision could take up to 2 hours in an 8-hour shift. Nine nurses were interviewed in this study, all of whom were sisters, charge nurses or more senior grades. Nurses supervised house officers in three main areas. First, the senior nurses often checked the dosages and drugs that house officers had prescribed; second, some of the nine nurses insisted that all house officers should be accompanied for all of their first practical procedures; and third, senior nurses tried to ensure that they accompanied the doctor when difficult news had to be communicated to patients. This obviously has resource implications but, more importantly, is unacknowledged work, which is invisible.

Power and nursing

In any branch of nursing, the relationship between the patient or client and the nurse is important. This relationship is dependent on the trust that will develop when two people are involved in intimate procedures. However, no matter how equal the partnership is, it would be naïve to ignore the power dynamics of the relationship, even if that varies over time. Where a situation occurs in which one person is feeling vulnerable, through a perceived loss of control because of illness, the other (the nurse) tries hard not to abuse that trust. During this period, nurses may perform certain techniques or use their knowledge and skills to enable the patient/client to become autonomous and independent of the nurse. However, when one person cares for another and therefore gives something to the receiver of care, that may unbalance or skew the relationship. This is because only one person is sharing his or her vulnerability. It could be argued that the relationship between the patient/client and the nurse will never be an equal partnership because of professionalism and the assumed boundaries that constrain professionals' own behaviour. Professionals are not expected to disclose personal information about themselves, which thus makes the sharing relationship inevitably unbalanced.

It would appear that, while nurses may have some control over the care of their patients, they have little managerial and organisational control. What little control they do have over other professions is not theirs by right; therefore they do not possess legitimate authority. Walby *et al.* (1994) argued that nurses will have to develop their own knowledge base to claim legitimate independence. Latterly, nursing theorists have made caring the focus of that knowledge development (Watson 1985). However, it is debatable whether nurses can really monopolise caring and claim it for their own. Other health and social care professionals also care about their patients and clients. The real difference between nurses and others in hospital settings is that nurses offer continuous embodied care, whereas other professionals only offer episodic direct care, although they may have a continuous responsibility as doctor or care or case manager. At the present time, the organisational control that has been lent to nurses comes by virtue of role delegation from other professionals and the organisation in which they find themselves working (Hearn 1982).

In conclusion, gender issues cannot be fully understood if the general social dynamics of the culture are not fully understood. Gender oppression cannot be overcome without some appeal to and support from legislation. Awareness of equal opportunity issues within the NHS has been raised over the past decades, and initiatives for promoting women's interests have begun. However, those initiatives do not actually change the nature of an organisational culture; it may be argued that they simply help women to fit into it.

During this chapter, various theoretical viewpoints have been explored. Whereas gender-neutral and excluding theories of power need to embrace the issue of gender in any future analysis, it now seems reasonable to jettison the emphasis on gender attributes and to discuss gender relations. Gender and power are interwoven. Within nursing, the invisibility of much of nurses' work is a pivotal axis for those concepts. Wherever nursing is, gender relations are present,w and it is important to understand how and

4 Elitism in nursing

Gill Mowforth

Introduction

This chapter will examine issues of élitism within nursing, attempt to explain certain élitist phenomena that have developed in nursing over the past 30 years and review possible connections between élitism and technology. The chapter will explore the topic only in relation to nursing in the United Kingdom, thus acknowledging the importance of certain historical traditions that permeate and layer nursing culture here but may not be relevant elsewhere. This is an exploratory, even somewhat tentative, chapter because there has been a very real absence of this topic in the nursing literature. Hence the chapter is reflective in nature and draws on personal nursing experience as well as social theories and theorists in order to illustrate certain aspects of the very complex subject of nursing.

The concept of élitism within nursing may seem somewhat paradoxical on first impressions. Nurses are rarely seen as an élite. Elitism within nursing, however, can be present in many guises, sometimes unspoken, sometimes assumed. Definitions and characteristics of élitism and élites and how they may be manifested within nursing are two main areas that will be reviewed within the chapter.

Status and élite theories

Weber, a sociologist writing in the early part of this century, rejected many of Marx's views on collective class identity based on shared interests and did not agree that class was the only basis for group-forming alliances. Weber believed that group formation on the basis of distinctions in social power – status – was more influential (Weber 1948). For Weber, money was not enough to have status; status also derived from the way in which people lived their lives and their pattern of consumption. With status, Weber argued, comes social power, power to exclude others joining the status group. Patterns of exclusion can take many forms, and status permeates all avenues of public and social life. One of the most common exclusionary tools is the admission criteria to a particular group. Weber described this as closure, a process that is frequently demonstrated in certain professions and aspiring professions by raising the educational qualifications for applicants (see Chapters 2 and 6). It also manifests itself in more discrete groups and élites, such as certain schools, certain universities, army battalions, social and sports clubs and certain nurse education departments that may be linked to hospital training schools of the recent past. Today, with the amalgamation of schools of nursing into university departments, the admission criteria into nursing are dependent on other factors, such as the fulfilment of contract numbers. Academic criteria for nursing education can change to adapt to specific local economic demands. If there were to be a surfeit of applicants, then no doubt the admission criteria would rise. Admission criteria for nursing are titrated to the demand for places. However, educational requirements are not the only prerequisite to join a group; other groups may depend on cultural, religious or economic attributes. Whether or not such specific status groups can be described as élites depends, in part, on theories concerning the nature of élites.

Classical élite theory

In classical élite theory, power in society is seen as being monopolised by a small minority who exercise power over the majority through the functions of the state. Elite theory concentrates on how people are governed. At the beginning of the twentieth century, two of the main thinkers and developers of classical élite theory were Vilfredo Pareto and Gaetano Mosca. They both described élite rule as inevitable and saw the rule of a minority over the majority as being unaffected by economic forces that Marx saw as responsible for class and class divisions. Pareto (1963) and Mosca (1939) both argued that it was superior personal qualities of the individual that made up the élite character, although they did not agree about the nature of those superior qualities. Pareto thought that the characteristics of élites were constant throughout history, while Mosca argued that they varied from society to society. Elite theorists often described the ruled majority as apathetic and uninterested in the important issues of the day, an unorganised and fragmented mass compared with the united and cohesive ruling minority. Mosca could see the advantage of democracies having 'open' élites, allowing various groups to be represented, but he regretted that the vote was extended to all members of society. He would have preferred to see the vote confined only to the middle classes. Pareto believed that élites became soft through the privileges of power and through a tendency for an élite to become decadent, thus ensuring its demise; another élite would rise to take its place. This he described as a circulation of élites.

Elite theory and the power élite

C. Wright Mills, an American sociologist, writing in the 1950s, fundamentally disagreed with classical élite theorists as he did not see élite rule as inevitable, or indeed desirable. He argued that élite rule was based on the exploitation of the masses and rejected Pareto's view that there was only one prevailing ruling élite. Mills argued that there were a number of power élites but that they all shared similar or the same social and educational backgrounds (Mills 1956). These power élites comprised the military, the state and the major economic corporations. The élites intersected and interacted on a number of levels. The men who were in the eminent positions shared a similar social background, which encouraged an interchange of personnel between élites. It would not be uncommon for those men to move in and out of the top positions within different organisations. Mills sets out a very cohesive picture of American élites, while other authors, such as Budge *et al.* (1983), argued that there are a number of competing élites who are probably far too fragmented and diverse to be a dominant force in society and are often in fierce competition with each other. The examples that Budge gives are of government, where the power is not only in the hands of the Prime Minister and the Cabinet but within divisions of and among the same party. Latterly, in the 1997 United Kingdom general election, major schisms within the parliamentary party, within Cabinet and between Ministers and the Prime Minister meant that the Conservative Party could not retain power in the polls. The Civil Service can be seen as a further élite group that wields considerable power. Hence Budge would argue that the state is made up of fragmented élites, thus limiting the power of government and acting as a safety valve, constraining the development of a ruling élite. However, a more important question to ask is, how can a minority keep a majority subordinated?

Processes of social reproduction

Theorists adopting a structuralist Marxist view, such as Althusser, have written extensively on how ideologies entrap men and women in a subordinated position (Althusser 1970). Althusser argued that the state has a repressive function that works in the interests of the ruling class by using government, prisons, the army, the police, courts and the administration to maintain order through dominance. Ultimately, such 'repressive state apparatus' could resort to legitimate violence if necessary. Besides the repressive state apparatus, there were more subtle means that also consolidated the maintenance of the *status quo*. Althusser described these as the ideological state apparatus, which included the Church, unions, the family, law, education and the media. These institutions, according to Althusser, change in importance over time. Althusser has been criticised for an excessively deterministic view, denying the possibility that the working class may be able to exert its own power.

Other groups of theorists have explored ideological processes. Willis (1977) and Weiler (1988) have addressed ways in which education can legitimise certain groups by the language, knowledge and patterns of interaction that are considered proper and valued. Gramsci's (1916) work can also contribute to our understanding of processes through which élite groups maintain power (Forgacs 1988). Central to Gramsci's ideas was a concern with the various ways in which the dominant culture imposed its own concept of reality on all subordinate groups, some more subtly than others. He addresses this through the concept of hegemony and defines hegemony as a combination of views that are diffused by the agencies of ideological control into every area of daily life, imposing power and control. The difference between Gramsci and Althusser lies in their different emphases on determinism and autonomy. Gramsci supported the view that individuals had the power to contest hegemonic control, as hegemonic power is in constant danger of being resisted and contested by subordinate groups. Gramsci argued that hegemony can be maintained through gaining legitimate consent within a society and through compromises on the part of the bourgeoisie to take account of the demands of exploited classes. Gramsci noted that intellectuals often deputised for the ruling classes and implemented the process of social hegemony. They were often afforded the cultural prestige that was gained through the possession of ideas and knowledge, at least in countries inclined to fête intellectuals.

Dominant culture theory

Writing in 1983, Susan Roberts described nurses as an oppressed group, arguing that they exhibited certain characteristics that Freire (1970) and Memmi (1965), two anthropologists, had observed and identified when studying groups. Memmi's work on race and colonisation, and Freire's on the language of the oppressed, influenced Roberts (1983) to examine the implications for nursing. These two anthropologists, studying different groups and at different times, had observed how the rulers, representing the dominant, often élitist, culture, often looked and acted differently from the subordinate, oppressed group. However, it was also evident that the subordinate group tried to emulate the norms and values of the dominant culture and tried to assimilate into that culture. Roberts observed that, if the assimilation was successful, the subordinate group became marginalised as their cultural identity frequently became obscured and invisible, which is often a consequence of an act committed by the subordinate group rather than by the dominant culture. This can sometimes lead to the destruction and loss of confidence of that marginalised group, through a process that Roberts described as horizontal violence, that is, violence or destruction meted out from within the same group against itself. Roberts found resonances with nursing today; although nursing is often classed as a homogeneous group, it is frequently fragmented in its vision.

The role of science and technology in élitism in nursing and health care

While acknowledging that nursing as an occupation does not follow the classical élite model, observation and experience suggest that there are horizontal and vertical élites within different specialities and across the various branches of nursing. Within that viewpoint, it is difficult, if not impossible, to detach the study of élites from the analysis of class structure. Elites in nursing seem to have developed alongside the societal value placed on the bio-medical model and its outcome and on the medical profession. Why this has occurred is unclear, but it may have something to do with how society values science and technology, and how it attempts to use scientific and technological knowledge to control life and death. Death can be seen as totally under the control of doctors and nurses in a highly technological environment, which then gives power and status to those workers. Within the technological environment, the patients are often physically and acutely ill. Media portrayals of the drama of intervention when an individual is close to death create a certain frisson in the minds of the general public as death is not usually visible to the majority in this culture. It would be fair to say that death has the potential to hold a fascination for the general public, possibly because of its invisibility, although it is not now a taboo subject. Indeed, as Walters (1991) notes, much has been written about it.

Nurses have a special knowledge about death and dying, but, for some health care professionals, health care technology is accorded high status as a means of preserving life despite the fact that there has never been a satisfactory and comprehensive evaluation of care within high-technology areas (King's Fund Panel 1989). Currently, the scientific discourse is pre-eminent, and, according to Foucault, its claims to knowledge are in fact claims to power (Foucault 1980). Foucault argued that science has an ideological function. Knowledge that is gained through science may be used to sustain and maintain power balances between individuals or between groups (Cheek and Rudge 1994). While any occupation can claim the possession of a body of specialised knowledge, society has to be convinced that such knowledge has the possibility to improve the human condition before it confers status upon it. The superiority of some knowledge has been generated through the application of rational and objective methods of research and has been a critical element in granting Weber's social prestige or honour to some professions (Hughes 1990). The public perceive that they are dependent on the expert's knowledge, and within health care it is scientific and technological knowledge that is dominant. In some nursing specialities, in contrast, health care technology and scientific discourse may be less dominant, with consequent effects of the status of specialities such as elderly care, mental health and learning disability nursing.

Postmodern theory

Cheek and Rudge (1994) suggest that a postmodern perspective has much to offer nursing practice through undermining élitism by introducing themes that challenge the scientific discourse with its claim to objective truth. However, the term 'postmodernism' is problematic in itself as it is not a coherent set of positions, and attempts at a definition in most of the literature would appear to be a redundant exercise. Nevertheless, there are some recurring themes (Best and Kellner 1991). These themes centre around fragmentation instead of cohesiveness and heterogeneity instead of homogeneity. Postmodernism attacks the enlightenment ideals, challenges the scientific discourse and would wish to confront that which society has deemed natural. Postmodernism deconstructs tradition and offers a counter-hegemonic attack on a hierarchy of knowledge. Lyotard (1984) criticised social theories that emphasised the importance of class, race and gender, arguing that those categories were too reductionist to be of use. Postmodernism follows post-structuralist theory in the primacy given to discourse theory, with different discourses striving for hegemony. These theories need some careful investigation and some wariness on the part of the spectator. While postmodernism claims to be anti-élitist, for some emerging professions who have just found their voice and language it could prove to be silencing, despite its enabling potential: silencing because of the deconstruction of the scientific discourse, and enabling because it allows for the possibility of other paradigms becoming equally important.

Nursing and élitism

One of the paradoxes of nursing is that, while it is an essential element of the delivery of health care, it is often marginalised when major decisions are made (Robinson 1992, Walby *et al.* 1994), and that alone should exclude nursing from being described as an élite. However, there are groups within nursing, for example intensive care nurses and accident and emergency nurses, who have been described and perceived as such by other nurses and members of the general public. A certain status is therefore given to those groups by others. Those nurses do not have full control of their area of work, but they do hold power within certain specialities.

To explore this concept fully, it is necessary to look at the past and at how modern nursing has developed within the United Kingdom. Nursing historians have frequently emphasised early individual reformers, giving them an almost mythical status, rather than analysing the issues in which they were involved (Davies 1980). Davies argues that nursing history then becomes a weak, personalised history that merely makes a good story. This Davies describes as a progress-orientated view and not an analysis into the whys and hows of the decision making process. It is also important to explore the context in which those accounts were written – to ignore that is to ignore history (Godden *et al.* 1993). Adult nursing in the nineteenth century was heavily influenced by both Church and army, which both used hierarchical systems to organise large groups of people. Hierarchies have a way of silencing challenges and inhibiting debate (Hugman 1991) by controlling the use of resources and defining what is appropriate and inappropriate knowledge, and when subordinates should share in that knowledge.

As a consequence of Nightingale's work in the Crimea and the myths that surrounded her when she returned to Britain, she was able to set up a training school for nursing at St Thomas' Hospital in London. This pioneered the training of general nurses within the United Kingdom, which led to other schools being established in hospitals in which the training of doctors also took place (Abel Smith 1968). These early accounts of nursing exclude other branches of nursing's history and are really simply histories of adult nursing. The fact that the Nightingale school was sited at St

Thomas' inevitably led to the view that the most prestigious option was to train in a London hospital. That view persisted until the amalgamation of various schools of nursing in the 1980s to form Colleges of Health. This élitism was unspoken, but it related to the way in which the accepted reputation of the particular hospital reflected on nursing. Nurse training schools took full advantage of this in terms of recruitment and closure. When Nightingale started the first training school, she intended that others would follow suit, with hand-picked women to act as matrons. These women were all from the middle and upper classes, so a convergence of class, gender and élite attitudes was set in place. These attitudes were transmitted to nurses within their training programme. Nightingale was an ideologue and imposed her not inconsiderable power and authority on modern nursing. Nursing as we know it today emerged from a medical space in the nineteenth century (Gamarnikow 1978), and that pattern has repeated itself whenever doctors wished to discard an aspect of their work. This has led to the extended and latterly to the expanded role of the nurse (UKCC 1992a). A change from the extended to the expanded role has certainly been precipitated by the reduction in junior house officers' hours within hospitals. Nurses have traditionally filled those spaces and, because of this, have often exceeded the scope of their official job description and responsibility. This excess has often crept into the domestic work of nursing.

Perry (1993), with others, argues that nursing is not complementary but subordinate to medicine. Walby *et al.* (1994) reason that nurses have been conducting health care for a very long time but have not yet regained control over the creative and qualitative aspects of their work. Although clinicians have delegated tasks, Walby *et al.*'s research suggests that managers have been tardy in allowing nurses to carry out certain procedures. It can be argued that, if nurses do undertake paramedical tasks, remuneration should follow, but Walby *et al.* argue that managers want and need to keep nursing costs down. These arguments mainly relate to nursing in the adult acute nursing sector, and readers of the nursing literature could be forgiven for perceiving that technical processes are given a high priority, to the exclusion of such branches as learning disability and mental health. This can then lead to elevations of certain skills over others. The hegemony of technology within tertiary sectors of care sometimes obscures the qualitative aspects of health care that are required by various client groups who do not necessarily have solely a physical illness. Technological care and its associated epistemology attracts more funding and human resources in order to deliver that care. The relationship of élitism to the amount of technological care becomes more evident when it is granted a certain status by other nurses, clinicians, the public and the media. The dominance of technology can influence health care policy to the exclusion of the other factors when health policy decisions are made at government level. It is arguable whether this is entirely beneficial:

> there is endless talk about moving resources from hospitals into the community, about boosting neglected primary health services. Yet high tech tertiary services and hospitals continue to dominate the political priorities.
>
> (Pole 1996: 7)

Technological care dominates, not only the political priorities and ultimately the funding, but also the media. Where there are advances in medicine, this often means more surveillance of the individual, which doctors then delegate to adult acute nurses in high-technological areas. More nurses are required to monitor, interpret and report any significant change. It is this interpretation which is an important aspect of élites because they claim the knowledge to be able to interpret in order to be seen as experts (Cheek and Rudge 1994). Lawler (1991) offers further insights into why technical skills are thought to be more élitist. Basic skills often denote dirty tasks, while technical care often describes clean work. Dirty tasks are limited to the physical aspects of the body and are associated with, as Lawler identifies, nurses' and society's taboos. Technical care implies some objectifying of the body and hence distancing from taboos.

However, this does not altogether explain the popularity of high-technology areas as nurses' workplaces. Nurses within high-technology areas can be as much concerned with the subjectifying as the objectifying of the body. Adult nurses may be attracted to technological work because the ratio of patients to nurses is very clearly identified and they are then in a position to practise nursing, which is a fairly rare phenomenon according to Davies (1995). Davies reasons that, because nursing has such loose boundaries and a variable mix of staff, it would not be possible to describe a group of nurses as forming an élite. Nurses' work lies on a shifting and dynamic continuum, with technical expertise and knowledge at one end and domestic work at the other. It is this that has prompted non-nurses to comment on and question the need for qualified nurses in some specialties in all branches. Even for nurses, the loose parameters of their work can cause tension and confusion as they have often internalised the implicit values of what Goddard observed and described as basic and technical care (Goddard 1953). This simple, straightforward analysis of nurses' work in the 1950s may have set the scene for the stratification of nursing skills. Naming some skills as basic inferred that the level of skill needed to perform them was much less. Melia (1987) observed that basic care has developed negative attributes, implies a lack of skill or importance and deals only with the physical needs of the person, while technical care denotes more advanced skills that are linked to advanced medical care. Within the adult branch in particular, it could be argued that a hierarchy or a stratification of skills filled the space left by the departure of rigid hierarchies within the workplace. Nursing has itself always been ambivalent about who should perform the basic and technical care. Basic care has often been designated to people with the least status, education and training, and this division between dirty and clean work offers nursing its own class divisions.

Elites are not healthy in nursing, or in other health care professions, because the specialness or distinctiveness that élite groups claim for themselves can be passed on to their clients or patients, and this can affect the ways in which nurses and clients interact. However, it will prove to be difficult for nurses to resist the domination of the scientific discourse because the structures in which they work will not fundamentally change unless nurses are in control of that work. Even then, it is arguable whether nurses would necessarily and automatically reject the dominant discourse. In an endeavour to unravel the complex web of élitism in nursing, we need to examine what is meant by the word 'nursing' in the text. It is seldom that there is a distinction made between the four branches of nursing, let alone the specialties within those branches. Problems of nursing are often discussed in a universal context, treating all nurses as a homogeneous group.

Nurses are not a homogeneous group, nor are they an isolated group within health care. Nursing needs to explore ways of raising nursing's profile without introducing élitism and ways of valuing nurses' contribution to health care that not only measure it against the technological environment but also include the affective domain. Some branches have already and for some years taken up that challenge, especially within learning disability and mental health nursing. Sources of élite power in the main emanate from medicine, as doctors have control over their own and nurses' work. Within nursing, there are a number of contributory factors that have an impact on the occurrence of élitism and élites, some of which are conflated but do appear to be centred around the particular work in which the nurse is engaged. Is it a technical or basic or intimate skill? Who else can do it? What special knowledge is needed to carry out that skill? What social honour is conferred by others? Should nurses be engaged in élitism in any case? Unfortunately, élitism cannot be dismissed as a distraction as it is ever present, albeit in nebulous forms. It has no place in modern nursing in any branch because it interferes with all interactions, not only between nurse and client/family, but also between nurses and other colleagues who may have less experience but not less intelligence, and this can be a real obstruction to a healthy learning environment. To try to dispose of élitist attitudes, one of the ways forward would be to understand each other's roles and each other's branches in more detail and to be able to use that knowledge in clinical practice in an informed way. If nursing wants to continue embracing the professionalising project, it will need to overcome the assumed and manufactured duality and opposition between technical and routine knowledge (Turner 1987).

In conclusion, this chapter has tried to convey how élitism has seeped into nursing in various ways and guises. It has looked at various theories that may have helped to identify the problems. The desirability of developing élitism in nursing must always be questioned since it would create and exacerbate divisions within the profession. My own experience suggests that most nurses do not feel that they are in an élite position at all, although they may agree that they work in what are termed 'élite' areas. It is time for nurses to challenge the scientific discourse, and in many areas this is already happening (Ashworth 1990, Wilkinson 1992, Parsons 1994).

Nursing has a propensity to embrace the scientific discourse, and this has led to a limitation of nurses' perception of the nature of illness. The most used example must be the nursing process, in which the emphasis in adult nursing (although not in mental health or learning disabilities) has been on the physical assessment. However, it is no surprise that nurses have formed alliances with that discourse because of the professionalising project. It is an alliance that brings strengths, as can the new emphasis on evidence-based care. It would be impossible to nurse entirely on intuition and experience. What is necessary to regain and maintain is the essence of 'being there' for patients and clients at whatever stage they have reached. If all nursing interventions had to have a measurable outcome before one embarked on them, that would leave huge schisms between the nurse and the patient. Nursing care is often difficult to measure, but that does not mean that it does not have a positive value for the patient or client. It might just be less visible to the observer. Postmodernist and post-structuralist theories are useful and are certainly a way of intellectually challenging the dominant discourse by offering positions and explanations from which to debate these issues. However, it is important for nurses to adopt a sceptical view of the discourses, be they from a scientific origin or from the humanistic model. The postmodernists do have a number of positions and are eager to sweep the enlightenment ideals of rationality and objectivity away. Unfortunately, what they leave is often an empty space, while discourse theory does lend itself very much to helping us to grapple with nursing's paradoxes and ambiguities. Roberts' work on the implication of oppression for nurses is useful when searching for explanations for horizontal violence within nursing, but it is also useful to absorb the concept of dirty and clean tasks when analysing horizontal violence. Hopefully, with continuing education, nurses will take their place in health care decision making, but with decision making comes the accountability of the individual. One major concern for the future is that hospitals will continue to dominate the health care discourse, even though the rhetoric, as always, is that more acutely ill patients will be nursed in the community. The pressure on GPs, local politicians and ultimately state politicians from families and the media will be difficult to resist. It could be just at the moment when community care is in most demand that acute care will become even more élite.

5 Nursing teams and hierarchies: nurses working with nurses

Margaret Miers

Introduction

This chapter explores power issues in nursing teams. It looks at ways in which leaders or managers of nursing teams use power and the ways in which power issues shape and constrain nurses' teamwork and nursing care. The focus of the chapter is nurses working in hospital settings, in general nursing. The limitations of such a focus must be acknowledged; it is not a reflection of the scope of nursing practice. It derives, however, from emphases in the available literature. Power dynamics between nurses in community homes or in community health care teams warrant closer review but have rarely been researched, perhaps because of the difficulties intrinsic to researching staff relationships in such settings. Researchers, either as participants or observers, have perhaps found it easier to gain access to the more public settings of hospital wards than to relatively private contexts in which nurses work together in the community. Nevertheless, the interest in nurses' work in hospital settings reflects both 'the hegemony of technology within tertiary sectors of care' (see Chapter 4) and the élitism within nursing that leads, as Mowforth has identified, to a failure to distinguish between branches of nursing, reinforcing the dominance of adult nursing within histories and analyses of nurses' work.

This chapter, therefore, reflects rather than addresses sociology's inattention to learning disability and, to a lesser extent, mental health nursing. Such inattention can be understood alongside the constraints and power dynamics within which nursing teams work. These are many and have been usefully explored in earlier chapters. Nursing teams work within a context of gender relations, of professional subordination, of a patriarchal organisational logic, of economic structures, of policy issues and of an ensuing marginalisation that makes much of their work invisible.

Nursing in a gendered world

As Mowforth makes clear (Chapter 3), an analysis of gender and power identifies ways in which nurses' relationships with other nurses are framed by a patriarchal culture mediated through organisational structures. Acker (1990) identifies a gendered organisational logic. Organisational hierarchies assume that workers have no attachments, commitments and physical or emotional needs that may impinge on the job itself. This leads to a privileging of masculine approaches and to the 'golden pathway' career adopted by men (Davies and Rosser 1986). Part of the gendered organisational logic involves assumptions about the complexity of tasks and their relationship to hierarchical patterns of authority and responsibility. Tasks delegated to a secretary (or to a nurse) do not necessarily confer status in an organisation if such tasks can be seen as remaining the responsibility of a manager or doctor. Cultural assumptions ensuring that masculinity is seen as congruent with authority lead to a marginalisation and invisibility of women's work.

Davies (1995) has linked the gendering of bureaucracy – 'inflexibility, its tendency seemingly to forget its own mission, its lack of regard for persons' (p. 56) – to the gendering of professions. Professional emphasis on expertise, derived from a formalised training based on science, can be seen as being gained 'by dint of a lengthy and heroic individual effort. This effort results in knowledge as a "possession" of the autonomous individual' (Davies 1996a: 670). Professionalism can thus be seen as 'mastery' over knowledge enacted in impartiality and impersonality. Such detached, competent and autonomous practice can be seen as being associated with cultural notions of masculinity. In reality, Davies notes, autonomous practice rests on the supportive and subordinate clerical, secretarial and, in health care, nursing work, that is itself gendered. Davies sees ways of organising both bureaucracy and professions as 'oriented to control and mastery':

> Both create hierarchical relations to achieve this and promote distance from and even disdain for their clientele. The application of expert knowledge, be it associated with office or the person, retains a mysterious character and calls forth deference on the part of the recipient. It is particularly important to note that in practice, the work can only be accomplished in the requisite detached and impersonal manner by dint of a great deal of preparatory and servicing work which is carried out by women. This work is rarely acknowledged or well conceptualised; from the point of view of the gendered professional ideal it is regarded as trivial or as 'support'.
>
> (1996a: 671)

It is within this gendering of organisations and of professional practice that nursing is marginalised and invisible. Within such cultural domination, nursing can be seen as oppressed and can demonstrate characteristics of an oppressed group in that the group itself takes on the values of its oppressors and colludes in the cultural processes that make nursing's strengths invisible. Savage (1995: 6) has argued that 'until recently, the potential of the nurse–patient relationship was highly constrained' both by the emphasis on the patient as a biological body and, in general nursing, through encouragement 'to maintain an emotional distance from their patients'. Menzies (1970) identified the task allocation system of organising nursing work as protecting nurses from anxiety by reducing their involvement with individual patients. Nevertheless, Menzies, in her research at a London teaching hospital, identified high levels of distress and anxiety among nurses. This was not just because of the inherently stressful nature of work, which regularly confronts 'the threat and reality of suffering and death' (Menzies 1970: 5), but also because of the organisational aspects of nursing work. Task allocation denied the importance of individualised nursing care, and managerial policies that regarded nurses as detached workers who could move anywhere led to a disregard for the importance of individuals either as patients or as nurses. Nursing, in seeking detached impartiality through hierarchical control and Taylorist work methods, could be seen as colluding with the masculinist projects of bureaucracy and professionalism, maintaining their own silence about the demands and potential of nursing care.

Nursing teams and hierarchies

There is substantial evidence to suggest that nurses themselves experience working in nursing's organisational structures – nursing hierarchies – negatively. In a small research project concerning diploma student nurses' perceptions of power, 35 respondents (63.6 per cent) referred to nursing hierarchies as illustrations of organisational power (Newall 1996). One student was very specific about how the hierarchy worked:

> 'on the ward – doctors only talked to Sisters, then Sisters only talked to F/E grades [qualified nurses] then the E grades told the D grades to tell HCA [health care assistant] and students what to do, then HCA told students again, then we all told the patients what to do!'
>
> (Newall 1996: 42)

Although such a hierarchical division of labour may allow a clear allocation of roles and status and, as a functionalist analysis would suggest, generate consensus, some students commented on the way in which the hierarchical organisation separated groups of staff and generated 'conflict over power between staff of different grades... as opposed to working as a team' (Newall 1996: 43).

Smith (1992), reporting on her participant observation and questionnaire research into how student nurses learn to care, illustrated the effects of a ward sister's authoritarian management style on student nurses. A sister's reprimand to a student in front of medical staff reduced one student to tears:

> The abrupt and impersonal way in which she handled the student's omission, and seemingly colluded with the doctors, made the student feel humiliated and unsupported. Under such conditions, the student temporarily lost both her technical and emotional confidence to care for patients.
>
> (Smith 1992: 73)

Smith found that students' own caring styles and capacity to care was affected by a range of factors over their 3-year training trajectory. The extent to which ward management styles recognised or repressed individuality was particularly important, as was the way in which the ward management style could recognise the student's learning role and offer the student personal support as an individual and as a student nurse. Smith found that, in general, students were 'incredulous at the lack of support they got throughout their training from either their teachers or their ward sisters' (p. 128). Smith's research demonstrated the importance of student support (or the absence of support) in the development and sustaining of 'caring styles and capacities that recognised and valued emotional labour as part of their work.' One third-year student expressed the complexity of learning to nurse:

> In nursing you have got so many relationships to form with people who you have never met before, who you probably don't like, you may not like out of work, under circumstances that are tremendously difficult. Often the relationships are short and sharp with hierarchy and authority and discipline somewhere mixed up into them, the learning situation as well. And the student who is trying to gain knowledge from this person, who she is trying to form a relationship with, when you add all that together, well I think you are bound to have chaos and I think you do have chaos. And so I think that in the nursing world as a whole everybody moulds everybody else.
>
> (Smith 1992: 129)

Smith's identification of the importance of hierarchy, authority and discipline in shaping personal relationships in nursing supports Lesley Mackay's research that began in 1986 and aimed to investigate 'the problem' of nurse wastage. Mackay is forthright about her findings. She is prepared to call a nurse a bitch, not an angel:

> Learners who speak out, ask too many or inappropriate questions, may be labelled cheeky or troublemakers... learners learn to keep their mouths shut and to do what they are told to do... almost all members of staff on a ward can tell a learner what to do. The learners learn to take orders and to see themselves at the bottom of the pile... They even learn not to speak out too loudly about bad practices as well...
> The learners feel isolated when they embark on their nursing careers, they want to be accepted and part of the team. Yet because they do have to 'bite their tongues' they know they only partially fit in. As a result they are likely to learn to distrust other nurses who appear to fit in only too well. It is not surprising that in such an environment, learners come to accept, like qualified nurses, that nursing is bitchy. By accommodating themselves to the hierarchical system and denying themselves as individuals, the frustrations of nurses can be expressed through bitching about colleagues. The way in which learners are treated ensures the continuation of this extremely self destructive behaviour amongst nurses.
>
> (Mackay 1989: 34–5).

Smith and Mackay completed their research before Project 2000 educational reforms either had been implemented or could have had much effect on nurse education and practice. Mackay viewed the likely impact of the educational reforms with some scepticism, observing that:

> many of the difficulties identified in nursing are likely to obstruct any real changes in nursing. Nursing is hierarchical, often conservative and there is a dislike of those who 'speak out'. The ethos of 'not rocking the boat' ensures that poor nursing practices are not addressed: reasonable complaints cannot be made and suggestions for change are received in silence.
>
> (1989: 181–2)

Evaluations of Project 2000 reforms, however, suggest that Mackay's scepticism may have been pessimistic. Maben and Macleod Clark (1997) report that 81 per cent of 78 qualified Project 2000 diplomates suggested that the course had equipped them with skills necessary to effect change. Managers and practitioners supported this view; however, 'the issue of "fitting in" when in the clinical environment was acknowledged by the nurse teachers to be as prevalent today as a decade ago' (Maben and Macleod Clark 1997: 58). All involved in the evaluative research identified that the patient was central to the philosophy of nursing, but the potential for change was seen as being limited by the structural constraints of the health service in the 1990s. Mackay, similarly, writing about a different educational system, noted the importance of constraints on nurses' actions: 'The world of nurses is simply a reflection of the wider society. But that does not mean it cannot be changed' (Mackay 1989: 184).

Oppression in nursing

Identifying processes of change, however, may depend on the clarity of the analysis of constraints. If the analysis of nursing work has been limited by its invisibility, it may also be the case that the analysis of nursing's problems has been similarly constrained by gendered processes that make negative images of nurses unspeakable. Angels cannot be bitches. As Mowforth identifies, however (Chapter 4), negative aspects of the behaviour of an oppressed group may indeed be applicable to nursing. Nursing's internal 'horizontal violence' may be explicable through an understanding of the processes of oppression.

Oppression can ensure that members of the oppressed group have views about themselves that are self-denigrating and self-limiting. They are views that have been gained through contact with a dominant group that may use negative stereotypes about the subordinate group to serve as a method of closure, excluding the oppressed from the privileges of the dominant. Nurses, for example, may have internalised the view that caring is natural and does not require intellectual and educational development. That is a view that is in the interests of the dominant group (men, doctors, educational élites), who perceive themselves as possessing valued intellectual attributes. Nurses as an oppressed subordinate group exclude other nurses who adopt different views and demonstrate intellectual abilities. Nurses who appeared to think about caring, or appeared to think at all, could be ignored and ridiculed by other nurses. Hence, perversely, the oppressed group attempts to protect itself by silencing and excluding a discourse that might enable other nurses to make a more assertive (co-operative, caring, thoughtful) contribution to health care.

Davies (1995) has argued that the lack of recognition of the importance and complexity of nursing throughout NHS leadership and management has contributed to the poor quality of management in nursing. She argued the NHS failure 'to acknowledge that there is a management job to be done' (1995: 165) led to a reactive coping style of management on the part of nurses, concentrating on ensuring that there were just enough staff to cope. Davies argues that the coping style of management increases isolation, worsens resource levels and leads to managers asking more and more of their staff (Davies 1992, 1995). In a gendered organisation, with gendered assumptions about professional power, oppressed managers oppress their staff.

Management styles

Whatever the origin of negative management styles in nursing, what is clear from all studies of nursing teams is the importance of the management style of the nurse in charge. Mackay (1989) found that the most valued attribute of a sister or charge nurse was 'being approachable'. Smith (1992) reported that the 'ideal' nurse or ward sister had a 'caring side'. Students saw the ward sister as the key person 'in setting the emotional climate of the ward. An emotionally caring climate made the student feel cared for and thus better able to care for others' (p. 74). Qualified staff modelled themselves on ward sisters they had known and admired, admired for competence, for organisational and practical skills and for personal involvement with staff and patients. As one ward sister said:

> I think involvement is so important rather than this hierarchy system where the sister made people so nervous that you were actually afraid to express how you felt about anything and you couldn't develop your own role because you were suppressed by her system.
>
> (Smith 1992: 75)

There is now considerable evidence that the hierarchical management of nursing teams is on the decline. Nursing literature follows management literature in espousing the importance of devolving power and responsibility. Senior nurses in many settings work with explicitly patient-centred models of nursing that are supported by predispositions to become emotionally involved with those in their care and to help and support colleagues. The positive effects of such explicit orientations are noticeable to colleagues, clients and research observers. Field (1984), in his observations of a general medical ward on which he conducted a study of nurses' experiences and attitudes towards nursing the dying, noted the importance of the democratic and 'permissive' leadership style of the ward sister, her role in supporting her team, facilitating interpersonal relationships and skills and mediating between nurses, patients and medical staff: 'Her leadership style and strongly expressed attitudes were central to the ethos of patient care enacted on the ward.' Field, as researcher, expressed his appreciation of the nurses, thanking them for their 'courtesy, friendliness and frankness. If I should die in hospital I hope it is on a similar ward.'

The importance of supportive patient-centred practice has been emphasised throughout the adoption of the nursing process and through debates concerning primary nursing. The Audit Commission (1991) report on the use of ward nurses stressed the importance of continuity of care as a means of improving nursing practice. Furthermore, more limited government support for the importance of the nurse–patient relationship came through *The Patient's Charter*'s endorsement of the named nurse. Such 'official' recognition of the importance of interpersonal skills in nursing followed nursing's own increasingly clear commitment to continuity of care and the belief that support is an intrinsic part of nursing. Primary nursing is the method of organising nursing care that most clearly seeks to offer individual continuity of care by a caring and supportive nurse. Savage (1995) has argued that managerial support for primary nursing was facilitated by the introduction of general management in the 1980s. While the autonomous, responsible and accountable primary nurse developed a professional relationship with the client, the ward sister acted as general manager for the ward, taking on new responsibilities for resources and budgets (Savage 1995). As Savage (1995) illustrates in her ethnographic research, primary nursing had the capacity to enhance our understanding of nursing care significantly but, in Savage's research area, could not survive the efficiency savings of the internal market.

Changing the environment of care

Savage's research looked at nurse–patient interaction on two medical/surgical wards, one adopting a system of primary nursing (Jones Ward) and the other team nursing (Smith Ward). Her interest was observing nurses' behaviour with patients and nurses' accounts of their emotional and physical aspects of care. Savage identified the notion of 'closeness' as an important element in any conceptualisation of primary nursing as opposed to other ways of organising nursing care. Pearson (1988) saw primary nurses' ability to establish 'close' relationships with patients and to use 'closeness', established through intimate personal care in the context of a continuing relationship, in a therapeutic manner, as a means through which nurses achieved successful outcomes. 'Closeness', however, is not a concept that has been well defined. Peplau (1969) described a professional closeness as being 'closer to the truth' of a client's dilemma, but writers two decades later have implied that the closeness sustained through 'being with' and 'being there' involves a more reciprocal intimacy between nurses and clients, an intimacy during which the nurse confronts 'the vulnerability of her own humanness' (Meutzel 1988: 107). Such reciprocity, which has also been described by May (1991), can be a commitment that nurses find difficult to sustain. Savage's research focused on the nature of 'closeness' in nursing practice in primary and in team nursing and on the support needs of nurses working with different modes of organising care.

Humour, non-instrumental yet non-spontaneous touch, and body posture emerged as three remarkable modes of communication on the primary nursing ward. Nurses prioritised spending time with patients and had organised the layout of the ward to ensure that paperwork was done at the bedside (there was no central nursing station). Nurses:

> made what seemed to be a deliberate use of their body, consciously sitting or squatting by their patients, rather than standing over them during any interaction. As a result, the scene at times was more domestic than institutional and more reminiscent of a private sitting room than part of a hospital.
>
> (Savage 1995: 31)

Savage notes that 'what appeared to be happening on Jones Ward was that nurses were manipulating stereotypical female roles – or the association between female and private spheres – in order to *challenge* the stereotyping of their nursing role' (p. 97). The female, permanent nurses on Jones Ward appeared to have introduced a new way of organising individualised nursing care in the face of hostility from male consultants through transforming the physical, cultural and emotional context of care, changing a public sphere into a private space in which women were more able to have authority. In the open ward, in which nurses had no private space, nurses were always on view and their bodies were always publicly visible as they cared for patients. Nurses used expressive touch and a casual and open posture to communicate physical proximity and emotional closeness. They thus transformed a public space into an environment 'in which events and actions were given meanings generally associated with the private rather than the public domain' (p. 92). The ward and the caring relationships had the characteristics of family relationships in a domestic setting.

Recognising how, on Jones Ward, female nurses were able to resist hierarchical and bureaucratic structures and subvert the (male) gendering of the workplace can illuminate the importance of space in other organisational modes in which nursing care is delivered. Traditional Nightingale wards provided opportunities for constant surveillance of staff and patients; nurses' offices provide staff safety and private space but also communicate difference and distance. The nurses' use of space on Jones Ward was deliberate, designed to support elements of nursing philosophy such as 'closeness', 'openness' and 'parity'.

In observing power relations on the primary nursing ward, Savage noted a group of more senior nurses committed to the ethos of primary nursing who appeared to represent a level of 'flattened' hierarchy as 'collective holders of power within a wider group that was committed to equality, at least in the nurse patient relationship' (p. 37). Nevertheless, if such a group had an inhibiting effect on some junior qualified staff, students and staff spoke positively about the ward, and nurses 'received support from across the range of ward staff'. Despite good relationships with each other and with non-medical professional groups, Savage was 'struck by a sense of invisibility in exchanges with medical staff'. Nurses' knowledge base appeared to have undergone a paradigm shift, but this had brought no 'corresponding shift in the power available to nurses' (p. 38). Doctors did not necessarily support primary nursing's emphasis on information about feelings. According to one consultant, this was the 'wrong sort of information'. Savage compared nurses' work and relationships on Jones Ward, the primary nursing ward, with those on Smith Ward, with its system of patient allocation.

In contrast to the primary nursing ward's visionary ethos, the patient allocation system of organising care represented a pragmatic orientation on the part of the nursing team. A main reason for the nursing team on Smith Ward to maintain patient allocation as an organising principle was the flexibility it gave to provide continuity of care when that was possible, but it also allowed a flexible and egalitarian allocation of workload tasks at particularly busy times. The staffing levels and workload demanded this, whereas Jones Ward, the primary nursing ward, was more generously staffed.

Whereas a main difference between the two wards was the use of the ward space and an accompanying use of bodily practices, such as a more open, relaxed posture on Jones Ward than on

Smith Ward, Savage found that the nurses' articulation of notions of care and of closeness did not differ significantly between wards. Nurses' expressed their understanding of nurse–patient relationships in a range of terms on both wards, some evoking notions of love as a prerequisite for care, others identifying closeness as a mutual acceptance, some articulating an understanding of different levels of communication. All nurses, however, 'spoke of care as a response to the physical *and* psychological or spiritual needs of the patient' (p. 55). Through exploring the notion of 'closeness', Savage has been able to clarify nurses' view of intimacy with patients. It is an intimacy based on a 'fusion of bodily and psychological domains' (p. 66).

Such fusion may only be sustainable in the context of staff relationships that provide nurses with appropriate support and in the context of organisational modes that allow nurses to provide care. We have already seen how nurses' hierarchical and horizontal relationships and interactions have hitherto denied individuality, creativity and care through the perpetuation of conformity, exclusion, fear and anxiety. Savage's observations of two different modes of organising nursing care found, despite differences in the embodiment of nurse–patient interaction and the use of space, similarities in the support needs of nurses as well as shared views of intimacy. Perhaps surprisingly, the closeness of nurse–patient relationships was not seen as a cause of stress, although a generalised sense of distress in the face of patients' problems was seen as a difficult feature of nursing practice. Nurses on each ward found an *inability* to provide what they regarded as appropriate care far more stressful than caring. Further shared sources of stress were relationships with medical staff and lack of resources, although the latter was more of a problem on Smith Ward, the patient allocation ward, than on Jones Ward, the more generously resourced primary nursing ward. Nurses on both wards found considerable support from their colleagues. Support was tacit, ill defined, gained and expressed non-verbally, as described by one senior staff nurse on Smith Ward:

> I don't think people necessarily have to say anything. You know when people are [noticing]; you can *feel* support. If you're in an environment where there is none, you're really aware of it. I think we've got a good combination here. There's very good support here, but I don't think it's

> anything tangible; I think it's just there. And should the need for it ever arise, then it would be there, more measurably.
>
> (Savage 1995: 116).

Such supportive trust between nursing colleagues may have been enhanced by recruitment procedures that allowed each ward to recruit staff who shared their working philosophy. Jones Ward could look for nurses who shared a view of primary nursing as an innovative mode of providing quality patient care, whereas Smith Ward sought patient-centred pragmatic and egalitarian staff, prepared to 'muck in'. The invisibility of colleague support may not be confined to intra-professional relationships. Walby *et al.* (1994), researching relationships between doctors and nurses, noted that 'much depends on the innate capacity of individuals to recognise when colleagues are under extra work pressure' (p. 99). To describe such a capacity as 'innate' can be seen as simply a way of removing the phenomenon from the realms of empirical scrutiny, which contributes yet again to the invisibility of the processes of inter-personal professional support. Walby *et al.* (1994) and Allen (1997) acknowledge the importance of 'rule breaking' or 'non-negotiated' boundary crossing in nurse–doctor responsibilities as part of good inter-professional relationships, 'provided it was based on trust in the competence of colleagues' (Walby *et al.* 1994: 115). Inter- and intra-professional trust is another notion that remains unexplored and invisible.

Pragmatism in nursing practice and nursing teamwork

Despite apparently similar levels of colleague support on Jones and Smith Ward, it was the nurses on Smith Ward who were better able to survive the prolonged and profound changes in the NHS through the development of hospital Trusts and a market-led health service. Smith Ward experienced diminishing resources earlier than Jones Ward, but eventually Jones Ward experienced change that transformed the physical environment and the mode of organising nursing care. Savage (1995: 120) records that:

> significantly, once nurses on Jones Ward were no longer able to practise according to their 'visionary ethos', their support needs not only

changed, but also went largely unmet. As a result, many permanent members of staff were thrown into professional and personal crisis.

Nurses who had transformed (regendered) the physical space of institutionalised care in a way that allowed professions to work in egalitarian closeness with patients suffered. It may well be argued that nursing as a profession has suffered through the decline in acceptance of primary nursing as a progressive mode of delivering nursing care. Yet Savage's work also reinforces other important, yet often unrecognised, messages in the literature about nursing teams. Nurses have also always valued colleagues who are skilled organisers of nursing work. As Smith (1992) made clear, the ward sister who was everyone's ideal was 'calm, kind and considerate, but also got the work done on time' (p. 69). Ward Sisters also identified good organisation alongside practical skills and caring for the well-being of individuals as characteristics of their own role models. James (1992) has also identified the importance of both the organisation and *organising* in care work. She emphasised organising as 'a vital but under-rated aspect of the daily labour of care' (p. 492). James uses the term 'organising' 'to convey the immediacy and purposefulness of the organisational and managerial skills integrated within direct day to day care by carers' (p. 493). She sees organisation as the link that ensures that 'the balance of physical to emotional labour is developed and maintained' (p. 494) both in the domestic and the public setting. James found that caring for the dying in a hospice remained constrained by hospital modes of organising labour because of the modes of organising physical care. The provision of physical care and the physical labour provided the framework within which social relations developed, partly through the allocation of staff to shifts (for example, the early shift) in which more physical labour was planned. James emphasises the importance of recognising the separate elements that nurses as care workers combine in order to provide care, namely organisation + physical labour + emotional labour, but she does not explore in significant detail how this is done. Nevertheless, her identification of the importance of each of the elements offers nurses useful concepts for the analysis of their work.

Literature on nurses' relationships with other nurses and Savage's work on nursing intimacy and the organisation of nursing work suggest that it is the balance and integration of these components that characterise the supportive nursing team and the caring emotional environment. Nurses care as they do the work. The work is emotional and physical labour. It is organised. Sometimes the organising is overt, oppressive and hierarchical, and ultimately destructive of nurses' capacity to care. Sometimes the organising is flexible, pragmatic and supportive, as appeared to be the case in some wards in Smith's study, and in Smith Ward in Savage's research. Occasionally, organising is deliberate, visionary and specifically designed to facilitate closeness. Savage found that, on Jones Ward, profound organisational transformations of nursing and patient space could sustain a professional–client closeness without cost to the nurse. However, changes in policy imperatives, resulting in reduced resources and a lack of wider organisational support, meant that individual idealism on the part of the nurses involved could not prevent disempowerment and personal crisis as the ward changed both physically and in terms of organising nursing care. These accounts of nurses' relationships with nurses and nurses' modes of organising nursing care suggest that it is the links between organising, physical labour, nurses' embodiment and emotional support that warrant further analysis both in understanding nurse–client relationships and in understanding colleague support and teamwork.

Conclusion

This chapter has argued that the analysis of nursing teamwork has been hindered by gendered assumptions about professions and organisations that have made aspects of nursing work and nursing relationships invisible and unspeakable. Although the traditional hierarchical organisation of nursing teams has been clearly identified in the literature, it was not until researchers sought to understand its effects on employment and caring trajectories of student nurses that the disempowering damage to individuals and the profession was acknowledged. However, if nursing has been mistakenly protected from acknowledging its own horizontal violence and the poverty of its own anti-intellectualism, it has also been passively yet persistently denigrated by the invisibility of nurses' work. The potential power of nurses' embodied communicative action (Habermas 1984) lies in the support that nurses are able to give to clients and colleagues. Nurses' fusion of physical and emotional labour through personal and team organising of individualised care are just two of the processes that underpin not just health care, but also the intricacies of successful domestic and organisational life. The analysis of the embodiment of these processes is just beginning.

Part III

Nurses and the health care team

6 Nurses in the labour market: exploring and explaining nurses' work

Margaret Miers

Introduction

Nurses are the largest occupational group in health care, making up almost half of the total workforce. In 1995 there were 421,000 nursing and midwifery staff out of a total health service workforce of 917,000 (ONS 1997). Numerical strength, however, does not appear to bring occupational power. Within sociological literature, it is the subordination of nurses in, and lack of recognition of nursing's contribution to, health care that has been seen as worthy of study (Ehrenreich and English 1973, Garmarnikow 1978, Carpenter 1993). In comparison with other professions in health care and beyond, individual nurses earn little, yet nurses' labour costs are high.

It is not difficult to explain nurses' lack of power in the labour market through sociological lenses. A functionalist approach would explain nurses' subordinate position in the labour market and in the work setting through their relative unimportance in the division of labour. Despite the organic solidarity (Durkheim 1967) engendered (an apt term) through the functional independence of doctors' and nurses' work, doctors' knowledge and skills are perceived as taking longer to acquire and as harder to replace than nurses' skills. Nursing skills, indeed, are not seen as specific to nurses. Students, unqualified assistants, families and clients themselves are all seen as taking the role of the nurse at times. For many years, nursing as a profession seemed content to see its own workforce replace itself regularly, with young female nurses leaving to care for children and failing to return. Replaceability, coupled with lack of autonomy over their own work through medicine's control, set limits on nursing claims to functional importance. A trait analysis of the nature of a profession suggests that nursing is a semi-profession, with dependence on medicine denying it full professional status (Etzioni 1969).

Professionalisation

A functionalist analysis of nurses' work and of the nature of professions may have influenced nursing's professionalising strategy to increase its power in the labour market. During the 1970s, the development of nursing theories fostered the growth of nursing's independent knowledge base. The implementation of the nursing process encouraged a recognition of nurses' own role in assessment and care planning, allowing later developments such as primary nursing to explore and extend the limits of nursing's professional authority (see Chapter 5). UKCC Project 2000 proposals sought to place the practitioner at the centre of health care and thus sought to enhance the status of clinical nursing practice. Moving nurse education into higher education can be seen as a process of gaining legitimacy for nursing's own systematic knowledge. Project 2000 reforms aimed to free nurse education from control by service demands and sought to change the educational culture that students experienced, thus developing questioning, rather than conformist, neophyte nurses (UKCC 1986). Educational reforms were seen as preparing practitioners for a new professionalised status in which nurses, using nursing and not medical models of care, would gain power and authority through a newly autonomous relationship with the client and through enhanced decision making abilities and opportunities.

It is probably the neo-Weberian approach to the analysis of professions in the labour market, however, that has had the greatest influence on the nursing profession's own attempts to improve nurses' position in the labour market. Sociologists, too, have adopted a neo-Weberian approach towards analysing nursing's professionalising strategies. Weber emphasised 'the kind of services that can be offered in the market' (Gerth and Mills 1948: 182) as a means of differentiating social classes. Thus occupational groups become professions through struggles to gain control of market positions. Such power struggles are effected through control over education and qualifications, and through the state legitimation of practitioners. Witz has argued that the professionalising projects of nursing and midwifery have, for example, been based on a dual closure strategy, denying full professional status to affiliated occupational groups with fewer, or lower-level, qualifications while at the same time extending their own professional remit to cover work hitherto within the control of the medical professions (Witz 1992). In abolishing enrolled nurse training and arguing against the indiscriminate use of the term 'nurse' for unqualified staff, nursing attempts to restrict access from below. In arguing for an enhanced role for nurses as nurse practitioners, nursing is using credentialism to pursue market closure from below and above.

Carpenter (1993) has argued that British nursing has experienced three main professionalising phases during which élites within nursing have sought power and status within health care. The first, the Nightingale era, he saw as a 'pre-feminist movement which sought to expand the social position of women within prevailing male definitions of their role' (Carpenter 1993: 117). The strategy was in fact organisational rather than occupational, seeking to create a relatively autonomous nursing structure, overseeing nursing tasks and the cleanliness of the environment within individual hospitals. A second, overlapping stage, initiated through the work of Mrs Bedford Fenwick, sought to improve the marketability of nursing skills through developing training and a scheme of state registration. Nursing's knowledge base was seen as involving both biomedical 'technical' knowledge, for example about the germ theory of disease, and the skills of the 'good woman'. Although state registration was achieved in 1919, nursing was not a united profession; the branches of nursing had separate registrations then as now.

Carpenter's stage three would be exemplified by the search for educational reform in the 1980s, culminating in the Project 2000 educational reforms (UKCC 1986). Alongside the demand for supernumerary status for students, the UKCC sought to place the registered practitioner at the centre of the division of labour and thus recommended one grade of nurse and the discontinuation of enrolled nurse training. Support workers, although seen as essential, were not seen as the 'business of statutory bodies for professional education at all' (UKCC 1986: 38), and it was hoped that a new term for a helper grade would 'put an end to the indiscriminate use of the term "nurse"' (p. 43).

It is perhaps too early to say whether the professionalising project, facilitated through educational reforms, is changing the occupational position of nurses in the labour market. The fact that nurses' real earnings increased by more than 50 per cent between 1981 and 1996 if working in the NHS and at an even faster rate in the private sector (ONS 1997) says something but does not alter nurses' relative lack of purchasing power. Sociology can, at least, help to identify the inadequacies in the professionalising strategy as a means of market control. Professional strategies are themselves constrained, as Carpenter identifies, by the contemporary social and economic climate and are enacted within existing social divisions. Emphasis on professionalisation distracts from fundamental issues to do with culture and with capitalism.

Nursing as 'dirty work'

A cultural analysis identifies nursing as 'dirty work', and, as Wolf (1996) suggests, in the majority of cultures, 'those who perform dirty work are soiled by association'. Despite the skill and sensitivity with which nurses may carry out nurses' (and society's) 'hidden work' with bodily functions such as elimination, and despite nurses' broad range of 'clean' and clinical work with medicines and administration, nurses' role as 'dirty workers' inhibits their status and recognition in many cultures. As Douglas makes clear, there is in many cultures a ritual separation of clean and dirty work, associated with the demarcation and separation of the sacred and profane (Douglas 1975). Nursing itself separates its 'clean' work with medicines, equipment and administration from its 'dirty' work with human bodies through the observance of principles of sterilisation, through physical separation of management and learning areas from patient areas and through status differentials between acute and continuing care (see Chapter 4).

Feminist approaches

Nursing has traditionally been women's work and as such suffers from patriarchal assumptions about women's work as being unskilled. Feminist analyses of nursing see a gendered subordination in the workforce as arising through complex and overlapping processes. Garmarnikow (1978) has identified the perceived analogy between doctor/nurse/patient and father/mother/child and the consequent low status of nursing that derives from linking health care with the domestic sphere. Expectations concerning women's caring role, expectations shared by women themselves, are part of the patriarchal culture that shapes perceptions, ensuring that, for many women, continuing to care, in domestic and professional spheres, is seen as natural and inevitable. Similar gendered expectations about authority, knowledge and intellectual thought have maintained patterns of dominance and subordination between male doctors and female nurses. Davies (1995) suggests that, as gender stereotypes become less rigid, analyses of nurses' lack of power and status in the labour market have become more sophisticated, although the importance of gender remains central. The processes that maintain nurses' subordination involve psychology, interaction and, as Davies argues, gendered organisations and gendered assumptions about the nature of professions.

Whereas patriarchy itself has curtailed (and still curtails) perceptions and definitions of skill and knowledge, nurses' educational aspirations also take place within a class structure that is peculiarly linked to and defined by educational success. In moving into higher education, nursing is seeking gains through a system in which it has always been an 'also ran'. These are issues neither nursing nor sociology has yet addressed. Class-based assumptions about the nature of skill, knowledge and intelligence are perpetuated through a higher education system that itself values abstract thought more highly than physical labour. Gaining professional legitimacy through the education system is not an easy project for nursing.

However, the professionalisers in nursing have always been in a minority. Habenstein and Christ (1955) identified three 'types' of nurse – traditionalisers who focused on the patient and were deferent to the doctor; professionalisers, who were skills focused and self-assertive; and utilisers, who saw themselves primarily as workers. Nurses have rarely analysed their position as workers and as employees. They have been more interested in the vocational nature of their work and in their claims to professional status and professional autonomy. So, too, have sociologists, for whom the extent to which doctors, managers and the state have controlled the professional aspirations of nurses has been of more interest than the extent to which these groups also control nurses' conditions of work. There has been an academic neglect of the importance of the utilisers and of the disempowering economic forces that control nursing labour.

Marxist approaches

A Marxist analysis suggests the *possibility* of power deriving from the numerical strength of the nursing labour force itself, but such a possibility would only be achieved through a recognition that workers share interests because of their relationship to the ownership and control of the means of production. Proletariat wage labourers neither own nor control buildings or equipment essential to production. All they own is their own labour. The considerable power of their collective labour depends on collective action or threat of action, which in turn depends on what Marx termed 'class consciousness'. Nurses can be seen as health care workers who lack control over the conditions and means of providing care. As with Marx's proletariat, if nurses' work is effective and efficient, it is not nurses themselves who gain any benefits from a reduction in costs. If bed occupancy rates rise, a reduction in costs allows more patients to be cared for by the same workforce. Nurses, however, have rarely used collective action such as withdrawal of labour to improve their own conditions of work. Many nurses would not see the deliberate withdrawal of care from their clients as an option they could consider. Collective withdrawal of labour, for example, was not on the agenda of the Royal College of Nursing until recently. The Royal College of Nursing's (RCN) no-strike clause remained as a symbol of its memberships' perception of duty until 1995, when nurses voted to give themselves the choice of strike action, if necessary, in pursuit of their own interests.

Marxist approaches to explaining variations in workers' power emphasise the dynamics of both the labour market and the labour process itself. Barron and Norris (1976) have argued that labour markets become horizontally segmented into the primary sector and the secondary sector. Primary sector jobs have relatively advantageous employment conditions compared with secondary sector posts. Full-time posts, permanent contracts with holiday and pension entitlements, are primary sector posts that bring them possibilities of increased responsibility and further training, allowing enhanced opportunities for promotion. Secondary sector posts, in contrast, are temporary, part time and short term. Barron and Norris argued that the dual labour market served the interests of capitalism by controlling the costs of labour and, furthermore, reducing the opportunities for collective action. Part-time workers and full-time workers do not necessarily see themselves as sharing the same interests, further reducing the likelihood of collective action to improve their shared rates of remuneration.

Nursing has traditionally relied on an extensive secondary sector alongside 'core' primary sector workers. Although the relative disadvantage of secondary sector work has been reduced by recent legislation giving pension rights to part-time workers, a rise in secondary sector jobs does save money. Bank staff and agency nurses play an important role in service provision. Such changes in work patterns have been encouraged both by the market-led philosophies of the Conservative government from 1979 to 1997, and by organisation and management theory. Atkinson (1986) has identified a move towards labour flexibility that involves two sectors: a flexible, multiskilled core group of workers, and part-time and temporary workers as a periphery. (See Chapter 7 for further discussion of Atkinson's work in the context of Fordism and post-Fordism.)

Marxist analyses of the labour market have also identified the cost-cutting potential of a 'reserve army of labour' that can be deployed to fulfil labour demands at particularly busy times. Women with childcare and domestic commitments have traditionally served as a reserve labour force for retail businesses over particularly busy times such as Christmas and the sales. Nurse banks serve as reserve labour. 'Reserve army' labour is cheap, since pay does not have to cover holidays and pensions. Any society has to pay for health care through either national or private funds. National revenue for health care has to be raised through taxes that limit the freedom of the owners and managers of wealth creating (profit making) enterprises. Hence the control of labour costs is a capitalist aim. Improvements in employment conditions add to costs. The growth of the secondary labour market and the maintenance of a reserve army of labour controls costs.

Davies and Rosser (1986) drew attention to the manner in which the mechanisms of the secondary labour market in nursing – part-time night staff, bank workers – served to disadvantage *women* in nursing's labour market. More recent concern has focused on the health service's treatment of staff from ethnic minorities. The deliberate recruitment of workers from commonwealth countries during the 1950s was a strategy whereby the 'mother country' saw workers in the colonies as a reserve army of labour. Employers' low expectations for such workers, the lack of opportunities for staff development and promotion, and insecure employment status have all contributed to restricted opportunities for groups of staff who are disempowered by the workings of the labour market. Commonwealth recruitment in the 1950s is now seen as a strategy that contributed to the development of institutionalised racism within the NHS.

Braverman (1974) has identified the labour process itself as a means of controlling labour costs, through controlling the nature of work itself. Braverman saw that it was necessary for capital 'to realise the potential of purchased labour power by transforming it into labour under its own control' (Thompson 1984: 68). It did this through management devising social relations of production that involved a division of labour based on systematic subdivision of work. The importance of Braverman's work was his emphasis on the potential for new technology to deskill occupations, concentrating knowledge about the overall process of production exclusively in management hands. Nurses' attempts to develop a range of skills in order to provide holistic care can be seen as being frustrated by the increasing complexity of health care and the number of professionals involved. It has also been frustrated by the increase, throughout the 1980s and 90s, in managerial control, a further strategy to reduce costs in the NHS. As Thompson notes, 'the separation of work into constituent elements reflects the necessary principle for capital of dividing the craft to cheapen the parts, providing the basis for the subsequent destruction of all round skills' (Thompson 1984: 68).

It is easy to see how nursing's professionalising strategy, with its attempt to enhance the skills and autonomy of individual practitioners, would flounder, given the capitalist imperative of controlling labour costs. With student nurses no longer part of the labour force, with enrolled nurse training ceasing and with health care assistants denied the title of nurse, much of the labour of health care would no longer be provided by nurses. Management definitions and divisions of 'skill' can align with cultural definitions of clean and dirty work. Unqualified staff provide the care, do the dirty work. In attempting to gain recognition for their skills, nurses have unwittingly colluded in the deskilling of care and failed to disrupt divisions between clean and dirty work. Changes in health care that derive from the emphasis on the control of costs and using market mechanisms to seek efficiency, implemented through the NHS and Community Care Act 1990, are further deprofessionalising care. With increasing day surgery and the emphasis on care in the community, clients and carers have become part of the health care team. At the very least, when families become providers of nursing care, client–professional relationships change (McLeod 1995).

Nurses may, however, through their changed educational preparation, have set up the opportunities to become reskilled as managers of care, as the staff with a monopoly of knowledge concerning the significance and hence the co-ordination of the care process and its mode of execution. It is this knowledgeable overview that is denied to the unqualified workers and family carers. However, it is the opportunity to deliver care that is denied to the registered practitioner.

Managerialism and professions

Nurses' dissatisfaction with the outcome would be no surprise to Braverman, for he recognised that the process of deskilling and of management control brought the conditions of alienation. Nurses are frustrated by their diminishing opportunities to nurse. Davies (1995) has identified this as the 'Polo mint problem', when, in Pembrey's terms, the practice of nursing 'drops through the vacuum in the middle' (Pembrey 1985). Far from feeling reskilled through their management role, nurses are frustrated and dissatisfied. Despite the efforts to improve nurses' position in the health care labour market and despite public popularity, nurses' professionalising project has failed to bring the expected rewards for the individual practitioner and has, apparently, failed to improve the position of nurses within the overall management of health care.

Within the context of the health care reforms and the managerial attempts to control expenditure, if necessary through the control of professional autonomy, this is hardly surprising. Nursing introduced its own educational reforms at the same time as the introduction of general management in health care through the Griffiths reforms following the Griffiths Report (1983). These managerial reforms could be seen as an attempt to improve the efficiency of health care through curbing the power and autonomy of the medical profession. NHS hospitals had hitherto had elements of three types of hierarchy – clinical-professional, administrative-bureaucratic and political (Davies and Francis 1976). Nevertheless, as Ackroyd (1995) argues, it was the consultants who exercised the greatest power and authority, and it was consultants' authority that was curtailed by general management reforms. These reforms were established by the government in order to facilitate the development of modes of estimating costs and expenditure as prerequisites for the development of an internal market in health care. Control of costs and expenditure was a management rather than a professional responsibility. Thus, while nursing sought to emulate the medical profession's strategy, by revaluing the importance of clinical practice through educational reform and through introducing the clinical grading system in 1988, general management challenged professional and clinical autonomy. Nevertheless, as Lorbiecki (1995) has illustrated, strengthening management in NHS Trusts involved effective collaboration with clinicians, largely through the development of clinical directorates and the involvement of consultants in management, creating perhaps, as Freidson (1984) recognises, internal stratification within the medical profession, some having more administrative power than others. Ackroyd sees nurses as undoubtedly the losers through the effects of general management. Nursing lacked the tradition of autonomous professional practice that enabled medicine to withstand the attentions of cost-cutting managers. In addition, as the largest occupational group, nurses will be the main targets for wage control.

Ackroyd (1995) notes that the functional importance of nurses within the organisation of the hospital prior to the Griffiths reforms has been neglected. He argues that the organisation of hospitals was characterised by a pattern of organisation described by Klein as a 'producers co-operative' in which doctors and nurses 'effectively co-ordinated and directed the organisation in which they worked' (Ackroyd 1995: 224). The practical activity of the nurses, their clinical role and their organisational and managerial activities were crucial. Nurses moved patients, organised supplies and co-ordinated the work of other professionals. In contrast to the feminist emphasis on nurses' subordinate role in relation to doctors, Ackroyd celebrates doctor–nurse co-operation. Nursing has indeed failed to pay due account to the importance of their organisational and team management skills. In shedding their domestic tasks and 'housekeeping' function, they have not lost their role as the professional group that provides continual care, but they have failed to ensure that this is a strength. This lack of attention to some key skills is explicable mainly through an understanding of the hierarchical approach to the management of the service. Matrons and ward sisters maintained the centrality of their position within the organisation largely through the control of information and of the intricacy of personal communications and inter-professional relations. They provided what the doctors wanted, perhaps what the patients needed, and they looked after their own nurses. However, they controlled their own staff through control over decision making and access to knowledge and information. Senior staff kept their knowledge to themselves. Tacit knowledge, transmitted informally and probably highly selectively, probably helped to maintain a hierarchy and deference that have now often left nursing without a voice once managerialism became established within NHS Trusts and senior nurses lost managerial roles.

Lacking a role in management, nurses play no role in decisions concerning skill mix. Nurses feel that their jobs are vulnerable. Ackroyd notes that 'it is a salient fact that morale can be shown to be lowest precisely in those areas of hospitals, and among those staff, that are functionally most important for the hospital organisation' (Ackroyd 1993, 1995: 237).

However, as this chapter has already identified, arguments concerning functional importance are limited in explaining the nature of social organisation. Functional importance may indeed ensure the continued demand for nurses in the labour market, but such importance alone will not ensure a change in nursing's subordinate status. Critiques of functionalism show how perceptions of importance are themselves culturally and politically determined. Analysts and practitioners of nursing have their own biases when seeking to identify the nature of nurses' work. Emphasis on nurses' work outside the medical model has led to an exploration of nursing care as opposed to skills supportive in medical 'cure' work. Nurses' ability to engage simultaneously in emotional labour and practical labour has been identified by James as 'carework' (James 1992). Macleod (1994) and Wolf (1986a, 1986b) have explored the extent to which nurses 'perform sophisticated skills unobtrusively' (Wolf 1996). Some aspects of nurses' work, however, such as their work as co-ordinators of care, have been largely unexplored.

Yet it remains nursing's functional importance in the organisation and nursing's popularity with clients that remain the source of nursing's strength in the labour market. Nursing's functional importance derives from its interdependence with the medical profession, other professional groups and clients and carers. Nurses, however, have minimised the importance of their role through allowing their influence to be part of the doctor–nurse game, as Stein (1978) identified (see Chapter 7). Mackay makes it clear that, if nurses are to realise their potential through developing their relationship with *patients*, they must also see clearly their own passivity and deference in work performances in many hospital settings. Mackay comments that:

> the performances in which nurses participate act to reduce the confidence of nurses in their own independent action. Nurse training, nursing practice and doctor's behaviour towards nurses all play some part in the level of assertiveness and confidence displayed by nurses... Too often the performance is face-saving behaviour undertaken by nurses on behalf of doctors. It is face saving undertaken by the less well paid on behalf of the much better paid. Nurses' career prospects, their status and their power are substantially less than doctors'. Yet nurses have been trained to protect their 'superiors'. Nurses' socialisation ensures that, in effect, they are active in maintaining their own subordinate position.
>
> (1995: 358)

The complexity of educational, managerial and economic changes that are affecting all nurses makes it difficult to analyse the consequences of strategies to improve their position in the labour market. The decline in permanent posts and the increase in feelings of insecurity, despite an identified shortage of nurses in 1997, are trends that affect workers in many jobs throughout Britain. Such trends have been a means of controlling costs within a period of recession and a period in the health service when the Conservative government's (1979–97) determination to control costs through establishing an internal market had been firm. A dual closure professionalising strategy can be seen to have been partly successful (Witz 1992). Unqualified staff cannot take the title 'nurse' and some nurses are working in more autonomous roles within health care. However, if some nurses feel they have opportunities to extend their skills, they see themselves as working under increasing pressure, and many feel deskilled and devalued. Health care assistants as well as other health and social care professionals seem able to take over their work. Nurses feel vulnerable.

Yet it is difficult to see whether nurses' importance in the labour market has reduced significantly, and if so, why. Student nurses were always unqualified carers, always cheap labour, always dissatisfied, always stressed (see Chapter 5). Hitherto, the task-orientated nature of nursing care and the subservience of nurses to their own seniors and to the medical profession suggest that nursing itself was complicit in organising nursing work in Fordist efficiency to suit the health service bureaucracy and the demands of capitalism, as Braverman analysed. Some nurses, nevertheless, took an effective managerial role, not only over their own area of work, but also within the hospital itself.

Caines (1996) suggests they could do so again, through MBA graduate ward sisters becoming clinical directors, 'challenging for chief executive posts'. It is possible to see many social processes that could now be enabling for nurses if they are able to identify and explore their own sources of strength. Caines (1996) has identified these as the move towards a primary care-led NHS, in which nurses with nurse practitioner skills could become the focus of change, and the development of 'peripatetic nurse specialists as deliverers of care'. Acknowledgement of the role of nurse specialists would be legitimising the ongoing process whereby nurses exercise judgements through doctor-led protocols. As Wolf understands, nurses keep order in health care institutions by 'looking after potentially dangerous people and containing the products of infection' (Wolf 1996). They are the bridge that separates and links the sacred and profane, the professional and the dirty worker.

7 Working with doctors

Sam Porter

Introduction

The occupation that nurses work most closely with is probably that of medicine. This chapter will look at how power affects this relationship. It will begin by attempting to describe the form that power relations between nurses and doctors take, noting that this is very variable. It will then go on to discuss some of the explanations that have been put forward about those relations. It will start by looking at explanations that concentrate on the market position of different occupations. Sociologists taking this approach are often highly influenced by the writings of Max Weber. The next approach to be discussed is that of feminism, which argues that gender, specifically the different gender balances within nursing and medicine, plays a crucial part in determining the relationship that exists between these occupations. Finally, those explanations which emphasise the important influence that wider economic structures have upon the position of occupations are addressed. The effect of the development of more flexible work patterns will form the kernel of this discussion.

Describing nurse–doctor relations

The first thing to ascertain when discussing power relations involved in working with doctors is, what form do those power relations take? There are at least four answers to this question.

The first interpretation of nurse–doctor power relations is that almost all the power is stacked in favour of doctors, leaving nurses in an extremely subservient role. A prime example of this position can be found in Eliot Freidson's *Profession of Medicine* (1970), in which he describes nursing as a 'paraprofessional occupation'. He argues that paraprofessional occupations:

> are clearly in a markedly different position than is medicine, for while it is legitimate for them to take orders from and be evaluated by physicians, it is not legitimate for them to give orders or to evaluate physicians. Without such reciprocity we can hardly consider them equals to physicians.
>
> (1970: 76)

We can see that, for Freidson, nursing occupies a very lowly position indeed, having no opportunity to influence the actions of doctors while being expected to acquiesce to medical orders. This rather black-and-white portrayal of nursing subservience is not shared by all commentators.

One such commentator is Leonard Stein, who has argued in his seminal paper 'The doctor–nurse game' (1978), that power relations between nurses and doctors are considerably more complex than might at first be imagined. Stein argued that the total subservience of nurses was only an appearance and that, while their contribution was hidden, nurses were in fact deeply involved in decision making processes about care.

Stein observed that because doctors are involved in life and death decisions, they are under a great deal of psychological pressure. One of the ways they are taught to deal with this in medical school is to think of themselves as all-knowing. Of course, this facade would be shattered if nurses were to make open recommendations or comments about their decisions. The problem is that nurses actually possess a considerable amount of knowledge, not least because they spend considerably more time with individual patients than do doctors. Therefore, if doctors are going to make decisions based on the best knowledge possible, they cannot afford to ignore the resource of nursing knowledge. They are therefore caught on the horns of a dilemma: on the one hand, they have to pretend that they alone are knowledgeable about care; on the other hand, they are dependent on nurses' knowledge. The way in which this dilemma is surmounted, according to Stein, is through the playing of the doctor–nurse game:

> The cardinal rule of the game is that open disagreement between the players must be avoided at all costs. Thus, the nurse can communicate her recommendations without appearing to make a recommendation statement. The physician, in requesting a recommendation from a nurse, must do so without appearing to be asking for it.
>
> (1978: 110)

This is usually done by nurses making statements about patients' conditions that carry hidden recommendations for action. This allows doctors to co-opt the implied recommendations and voice them openly as their own. Thus, for example, if a nurse believes that a patient requires analgesia, he or she will not say this in so many words. Instead, the nurse will inform the doctor that the patient is in pain. The doctor will then appear to make the decision that analgesia is required and will prescribe accordingly.

The third interpretation of the sort of power relations that pertain between nurses and doctors was developed by David Hughes (1988), who argued that, given the right circumstances, nurses had sufficient power to be able to make open contributions to the making of decisions. In a study of nurse–doctor interactions in a casualty department, Hughes noted that the doctor–nurse game was sometimes played:

> But for much of the time nurses seem much less preoccupied with concealing their role as advice-givers than the 'game' metaphor suggests. Nurses, even while acknowledging the doctor's clinical authority, frequently offer advice on many aspects of departmental practice in an open and straightforward way. More rarely, senior nursing staff intervene quite bluntly to point out shortcomings in the work of certain junior doctors, and effectively take control.
>
> (1988: 16–17)

The level of nurses' openness in decision making processes depended on the circumstances in which they were working. For example, because the turnover of medical staff was far higher than that of nursing staff, nurses, being longer in the department, had a far deeper knowledge of its customs and practices, which gave them an advantage over doctors who were not as familiar with the way in which things were expected to be done. It should be noted that, while circumstances could provide nurses with considerable power, doctors were still in a position formally to overrule them if they wished to do so.

Svensson (1996) has argued that doctor–nurse relationships can be seen as a 'negotiated order' (Strauss 1978) rather than a game. Like Hughes, Svensson found situational circumstances in which nurses' influence was strengthened and argued that a negotiated order perspective allowed microsocial interaction to be reviewed in the context of macrosocial processes. Interviews with 45 staff nurses from five Swedish hospitals identified doctor–nurse communication that was 'straightforward and open', explicable by a range of factors including the fact that the medical profession has been feminised (Porter 1991) and changes in nurses' educational socialisation (Svensson 1996). Nurses' practical work and nurses' knowledge of the patient as an individual were identified as key aspects of a new 'knowledge context' that increased nurses' ability to influence decisions. Nurses offered examples of negotiating with doctors around work boundaries in an open manner, although elements of Stein's doctor–nurse game still seemed evident. Nurses' work supporting doctors, including the introduction of new doctors to the ward, was identified as a resource in work-based negotiations.

Allen (1997), however, has criticised Svensson's analysis for its reliance on interview data 'which cannot necessarily be read as literal descriptions of an external reality' (p. 501) and also for collecting data only from nurses, thus offering a partial view of nurse–doctor relations. Allen observed and participated in the working world in a 900-bedded district general hospital for 10 months, researching negotiation processes and paying particular attention to 'members' talk'. Allen's observational data revealed little evidence of negotiations through talk but considerable evidence of 'non-negotiated informal boundary-blurring' in which nurses worked beyond boundaries, encroaching on doctors' work, in order to maintain the continuity and co-ordination of patient treatment, if necessary exercising independent judgement, including 'rule-oriented boundary blurring' (p. 511). It was the absence of negotiation and lack of conflict that seemed remarkable. Allen's study suggests that there may be considerable acceptance of nurses' influence.

The final conceptualisation of nurse–doctor power relations goes beyond the informal influence identified by Hughes. This involves nurses making formally sanctioned decisions about care that are independent of medical power. Central to this idea is the development of the nursing process, which entails nurses themselves identifying problems, deciding what should be done about them, acting upon those decisions and evaluating the results of the actions taken. It has been argued that the process, which gives nurses the power to diagnose problems and plan care, 'would give nurses autonomy and to a considerable extent remove medical constraints' (Bowman 1983: 10).

It can be seen that interpretations of power relations between nurses and doctors range from seeing nurses as totally subservient to their medical masters, to regarding nursing as an autonomous occupation with its own formally sanctioned decision making processes. This is not to say that we have to decide whether one of these interpretations is totally correct while the others are wrong. Indeed, Porter's (1995b) research indicated that, in different circumstances, all of these permutations of power are involved in nurse–doctor relations. He noted that there is some evidence to suggest that the nature of power relations has been developing in nurses' favour. During the Nightingale era, reflecting women's position in society, female nurses were in a position of extreme subordination in relation to their male medical colleagues (Gamarnikow 1978). However, over time, they have managed to attain ever greater degrees of autonomy, although attempts such as the nursing process to gain formal independence for nurses have not yet been completely successful. Moreover, nurses have not totally escaped from the shadow of severe power differences that existed during modern nursing's formative period (Dingwall and McIntosh 1978). For these reasons, the nature of power relations with doctors vary greatly, depending on the circumstances and people involved.

Explaining nurse–doctor power relations

It might be thought that the differential access to power enjoyed by doctors and nurses is entirely appropriate and unremarkable. Such an assumption could be based on the observation that nurses and doctors are allocated different functional roles in the health care system. The doctor's role revolves largely around diagnosis, prescription and treatment, while, notwithstanding the nursing process, the nurse's role is largely to assist with treatment and to provide care. While the balance between the two occupations may have shifted over the years, enabling nurses to have the kind of informal input described by Hughes (1988), it could be argued that this general formula for the division of labour between nursing and medicine still stands for the very good reason that it works. Doctors' training equips them to do different sorts of task than does nurses', in that the information imparted to medical students is more extensive and the skills taught to them more technically challenging. Given the knowledge that they have about the workings of the human body, it is only natural that they are the people entrusted to make major diagnostic and prescriptive decisions, which in turn often determine the sorts of action that nurses should be taking. In short, it might be contended that doctors have autonomy over their own actions and a great deal of influence over nurses' actions because they possess superior knowledge; as demonstrated through their possession of 'superior' educational qualifications.

Weberian explanations

Sociologists are intrinsically suspicious of claims that differences in power can be justified by recourse to functional reasons. Indeed, the use of educational certification as a means to restrict entry to privileged occupational positions was subjected to scathing attack by Max Weber:

> Such certificates support their holders' claims... to monopolize social and economically advantaged positions. When we hear from all sides the demand for an introduction of regular curricula and special examinations, the reason behind it is, of course, not a suddenly awakened 'thirst for education' but the desire for restricting the supply of these positions and their monopolization by the owners of educational certificates.
>
> (1948: 241)

Weberian scholars have argued that this was the route taken by the classical professions such as medicine to attain the privileged social position that they came to enjoy (see, for example, Parry and Parry 1976). Indeed, these professions took the process a further, crucial stage by securing the blessing of the state for their exclusionary tactics (Parkin 1979). By getting the state to accept that only those who had attained appropriate educational credentials could practise as a doctor, medicine attained a legal monopoly over many aspects of health care. This monopoly delivered far more than the autonomy of self-regulation; it also gave medicine the power to control other occupations, such as nursing, which worked with it (Freidson 1970). This was achieved by securing a monopoly over diagnosis and prescription. Because all actions stem from diagnosis and subsequent prescription, the diagnostician enjoys a unique position of authority in relation to both clients and allied occupations (Johnson 1972). These strategies, which attempt to create boundaries in order to maintain the privileges of a particular group, are known as strategies of *social closure*.

This Weberian portrayal of social closure might all sound very cut and dried, with medicine enjoying a position of unassailable authority in the health care division of labour. However, as we have already seen, this interpretation of nurse–doctor power relations has been contested by commentators who see nursing as enjoying greater autonomy than this model would suggest. It could be argued that conceptions like Freidson's (1970) of the lowly position of the 'paraprofessional' occupations fails to take account of the fact that nurses have also been playing the game of social closure. Mrs Bedford Fenwick's campaign around the turn of the century to introduce a legally sanctioned register of nurses might be seen in this light as a strategy aimed at enhancing the occupational status of nursing through restriction of access to its ranks to those with appropriate qualifications (Witz 1992). Similarly, as we have already seen, the development of the nursing process, which includes nursing diagnosis and planning, challenges the medical monopoly over diagnosis and prescription. Obviously, the story is more complicated than Weberian portrayals of the monopolisation of power and autonomy by the established professions can account for.

Feminist explanations

While seeing much merit in Weberian analyses of power, which attempt to uncover the mechanisms whereby occupations gain and maintain market control over the services that they provide by means of monopolisation and social closure, feminists contend that they suffer from gender blindness (see, for example, Crompton 1987). This is a significant gap, given that the most striking difference in the composition of nursing and medicine is that of sex, medicine historically being a male occupation, while nursing remains numerically dominated by women. Indeed, Gamarnikow (1978) has argued that, from their formation as modern occupations in the nineteenth century, the relationship between these two groups has been defined by gender inequalities:

> This ideological reconstruction of interprofessional relations and their transformation into male–female relations operated by representing the nurse–doctor triad as essentially homologous to the family structure. Thus doctor–nurse relations came to be seen basically as male–female relations and the patient became the 'child'. The equation... provided the space for turning nurses into 'mothers' and doctors into 'fathers'.
>
> (1978: 110)

According to Garmarnikow, doctors, being invested with the 'rule of the father', had the right to decide who should be regarded as a patient and what should be done to them, while nurses were expected to adopt a mothering role that involved doing the bidding of the doctor/father and caring for the patient/child. While power relations may have shifted over time in favour of nurses, it would be unwise to underestimate the durability of gender inequality that exists between the occupations. As Dingwall and McIntosh note:

> The Victorian ethos of male superiority reinforced the nurses' deferential attitudes to doctors far into the twentieth century, and the idea of a colleague relationship is a relatively new concept.
>
> (1978: 107)

Reflecting these insights, feminists argue that, if accounts of power relations between the occupations of nursing and medicine are to be persuasive, they must take account of the crucial issue of gender. Thus, for example, Witz (1992) argues that, in order to rectify the 'androcentric bias' of traditional Weberian accounts, we need to accept that occupational power relations are too complex to be explained by a fixed and general model of professional power based on that enjoyed by 'male' professions such as medicine. Developing the work of Parkin (1979), she asserts that occupations such as nursing and midwifery have been involved in what is termed a *dual closure strategy*. The strategy is described thus because it not only involves challenging the powers of medicine, but also entails nurses engaging in their own strategies of occupational closure. For example, in Britain nursing is governed by an independent body dominated by nurses – the UKCC. The UKCC has the power to maintain a register, to decide on the qualifications that are required to enter that register and to decide who is fit to be on the register. There are two ways in which to look at the occupational power that this autonomy brings with it. On the one hand, it means that the internal control of the occupation is no longer in the hands of doctors – Witz calls this side of the dual closure strategy *usurpation*, in that it involves usurping control from medicine. On the other hand, nurses now have the power to keep out those who are not deemed acceptable to the occupation – this is termed the strategy of *exclusion*. A controversial example of occupational exclusion can be found in rule 18 of the 1983 Statutory Instruments of the Nurses, Midwives and Health Visitors Act, which states that only 'first-level' nurses are allowed to devise and assess care plans. Thus, nursing process care plans involve not simply the usurpation of medicine's monopoly over diagnosis, but also the exclusion of enrolled nurses from the privileges of professional autonomy.

Some feminists are deeply suspicious of the sort of professionalising strategies described above. They see them as fundamentally flawed in that they involve attempts to play men at their own game and are thus doomed to failure. As Davies puts it, 'an advance into the old professionalism is an advance into a cul de sac' (1995: 152). She comes to this conclusion because she regards professional ideology as being masculine in its cultural construction. For example, professional knowledge is gained by heroic individual effort. The knowledge gained is thus possessed by the professional and cannot be easily shared with others – professionals control and shape knowledge, and through this control people. Moreover, professional encounters are marked by an impersonality and impartiality that act to keep emotions at a distance. All of these attributes are very one sided in that they reflect what are culturally regarded as masculine traits, which are contrasted with what are seen as inferior feminine cultural codes that emphasise attributes such as connectedness, selflessness and emphasis on experience.

Thus professionalism, as the embodiment of masculine, indeed misogynist culture, reinforces power differentials between those in male-dominated professions and those in female occupations. Davies' solution to this problem is not simply to emphasise the importance of female attributes. She argues that, while it is important to identify and celebrate the differences of feminine cultural codes, this should be part of a project that does not simply reverse the value attached to cultural codes (regarding feminine codes as superior to masculine ones) but that attempts to overcome the binary opposition between masculine and feminine codes.

Thus, for Davies, the new practitioners will be neither distant (masculine) nor involved (feminine), but engaged. They will be neither autonomous nor dependent, but interdependent; neither instrumental nor passive, but the instigator of encounters in which solutions can be negotiated; neither the master of knowledge nor the user of experience, but the reflective user of experience and expertise (1995: 149–50). In sum, Davies sees the solution to the professional predicament in nursing neither in attempts to ape male professions, nor in separatist efforts that see women withdraw into their own spaces, but instead in 'the move beyond gendering and the power/passivity dichotomy that this invokes' (1995: 150). This is not to say that she is adopting a neutral position – it is only through the uncovering and celebration of the hitherto repressed feminine that such a state of affairs can develop.

There is evidence that nursing theory and practice are responding to the sorts of concern highlighted by Davies. This can be seen, for example, in the increasing influence of Schön's (1983) concept of the 'reflective practitioner', which involves a rejection of the traditional idea of professional as scientific expert. While such developments may well be having a beneficial effect upon nurse–patient relationships, the degree to which they have had an impact upon nurse–doctor relationships is less certain. The effects of alterations in the professional ideology of nursing are restricted by the fact that medicine continues to rely on traditional, masculinist notions of profession.

Before leaving the issue of gender, it should be noted that some feminists have argued that the 'ethos of male superiority' (Dingwall and McIntosh 1978: 107) that animates nurse–doctor relationships is reinforced by blatant misogyny. To put it crudely, nurses are often regarded by doctors and others as skivvies and/or sluts. In relation to the former, Abbott and Wallace (1990) have noted how nursing is often regarded as mundane 'women's work', much the same as housework, which is in itself seen as requiring few skills and little knowledge. In relation to the latter, Muff (1982) has identified the sexual stereotype that sees nurses as sexually permissive. She argues that the purpose of such stereotypes is to provide easy solutions to the complexities of human relationships. They:

> obviate the need for men to understand each woman (nurse) as an individual by providing categories within which to 'file' her, and to transform the women (nurse) into *his* ideal to make her more acceptable and accessible and to lessen his guilt by association. (p.120)

Unfortunately, it is not simply a matter of degrading stereotypes. Game and Pringle (1984) have argued that these sorts of attitude often result in sexual harassment. They argue that sexual harassment of female nurses is not simply a matter of sex. It is also about occupational power:

> Doctors exercise not only the power of the father but direct sexual power over nurses. Medical dominance is reaffirmed by sexual domination. (p.108)

In their research conducted in operating theatres, they noted that surgeons had the power to enforce sexual contact on nurses as part of the nursing duties, for example getting nurses to mop them or scratch itches on the pretext that they were gowned up. Nurses found this humiliating but felt unable to refuse. In this way, the occupational subordination of nurses was reinforced.

Economic explanations

While gender is an extremely important social factor influencing the nature of nurse–doctor power relations, it is not the only one. Another way of approaching the problem is to examine how these occupations fit into wider economic structures. One of the most significant debates currently being conducted in economic sociology concerns the extent of changes in the nature of industrial production. The debate hinges round what are known as *Fordism* and *post-Fordism*.

Fordism is named after the famous American car manufacturer Henry Ford. It refers to the process of mass production that he pioneered, which involved the construction of standardised products from standardised parts on a moving assembly line. Such a system reduced costs, first because the standardisation of parts meant that a large number of similar products could be produced, which led to economies of scale, and second because workers, located at specific points on the assembly line, did the same simple task over and over again, reducing the need for expensive skilled labour while further increasing production rates. This style of work was closely associated with *Taylorism*, named after Frederick Taylor, who argued that the most efficient use of labour was to work out scientifically the best way to perform a particular task and then train the worker to perform the task in exactly that fashion over and over again. Using these methods, Ford managed to undercut the costs of other manufacturers who could only turn out small numbers of cars, using skilled workers who performed numerous tasks in the best way they themselves saw fit. The success of Ford was emulated by other manufacturers to the point at which Fordism became the standard production technique in the industrialised world.

One of the problems with Fordism was that it was very inflexible, involving as it did the production of standardised products. As Henry Ford famously put it when asked about the choice of colours for his Model-T – 'any colour so long as it's black'.

Fordism is now being challenged by a more flexible mode of production, known as post-Fordism. With the development of new technology, notably computers, machine tools have become far more sophisticated and can rapidly be reprogrammed to perform different tasks. This means that it is now economic to produce small batches of more specialised products, enabling producers to respond rapidly to changing consumer demands and tastes. The other side of the coin is that consumers have come to expect more choice in the products available to them.

In addition to technological flexibility, there has also been a move towards labour flexibility. The new pattern often involves a division of the labour force between a core group that is multi-skilled, and highly flexible in terms of the tasks that can be performed, and a periphery group, which is flexible in terms of time, in that it is composed of part-time and/or temporary workers, and workers employed by smaller, subcontracting firms (Atkinson 1986).

To return to the relationship between nursing and medicine, we need to ask two questions. First, has post-Fordism affected the health service? Second, if it has, what effect has it had upon power relations between nurses and doctors?

The answer to the first question is complicated. On the one hand, there is much evidence that post-Fordism is having an increasing influence over the provision of health care. Certainly, the whole idea of individualised care can be fitted into this model. The central philosophy of individualised care is that clients each have their specific needs, wants and fears, and therefore require a customised package of care that can best deal with the specifics of their situation. A corollary of this is the expectation that decisions should be based on reflective professional judgement concerning particular cases, rather than on the dictates of routine.

However, the problem with post-Fordism within a health care context is that it takes a great deal of time and effort. There are very real pressures on health services to concentrate on quantity in terms of throughput, at the expense of quality in terms of meeting the more idiosyncratic needs of patients. This has led to considerable tension, as Walby *et al.* discovered in their study of hospital organisation:

> There was a contradiction between the desire for higher throughput typical of Taylorist management and a Fordist regime, and the patient-centred, ward based, cohesive interprofessional team more appropriate to new wave management and post-Fordism. If the patient, as consumer is the centre with individuated packages of care, then Tayloristic management is inappropriate. The tension between these coexisting logistics of organisation was evident in many issues in the hospital.
>
> (1994: 158)

How does all this affect the power balance between nursing and medicine? The answer to this question largely revolves around the degree of decision making power that each mode of activity affords nurses. A post-Fordist organisation of health care tends, because it places so much emphasis on the individual practitioners, to increase the power and autonomy of nurses, while Fordism and Taylorism, which emphasise mass production and the rote repetition of activities, tend to undermine the decision making capacities of nurses. A Fordist organisation of health care would include task-centred care, whereby a nurse would perform the same discrete task in exactly the same way on a large number of patients. Similarly, Fordist care would involve an authoritarian approach by medical consultants who would lay down very rigid rules about how certain conditions (as opposed to people) should be treated by nurses. In contrast, post-Fordist care would emphasise the importance of individualised care plans, along with forms of work organisation, such as primary nursing, that facilitate flexibility rather than uniformity of care.

All this seems to indicate that post-Fordism is a good thing for nurses in that it involves increasing autonomy. However, if we remember the distinction between core and peripheral workers that often characterises post-Fordism, we can see that there is a downside. While trained nurses with flexible skills may well be benefiting from the increasing emphasis on professional responsibility of the individual practitioner, the number of nurses within this category has fallen steadily, as ever greater reliance is placed upon untrained nurses. For example, in a single year from 1990–91, the number of qualified nurses employed by the NHS fell by over 5 per cent, while the number of unqualified staff rose by 17 per cent (Ranade 1994). As a result of this widespread change in the balance of skill mixes, an increasing number of nurses find themselves on the margins of employment, suffering from low wages, insecure contracts and poor working conditions. Even worse is the peripherality experienced by those health care workers employed by outside contractors, whose wages, terms and conditions often fall below the least generous offered by the NHS. From this perspective, post-Fordism can be seen as improving the occupational position of some while undermining the security of many others.

All the different approaches to explaining nurse–doctor power relations suggest that power relations are capable of change, bringing greater autonomy to some nurses. This process is facilitated by changing models of professionalism, by social closure strategies and by post-Fordism. The approaches and models outlined in this chapter will help us explore the detail and dynamics of change.

8 Health care teams in the community

Margaret Miers

Introduction

This chapter adopts a Foucauldian analysis of power in order to explore the effects of professional discourses on the development of health care teams in community care and to review the potential for nurses to play a significant role developing community health practice.

Foucauldian studies of health care

In Foucault's analysis, power is everywhere. It comes from everywhere, through relations, through ideas, through language, through practices. Power is a force that affects our perceptions, our identities, our behaviour and our beliefs. As Barker (1993) describes, in Foucault's work, 'power... is an aggregation of different tactics and strategies, and individuals experience themselves in relation to these tactics and strategies' (p. 80). Power thus exists in and through relationships, interaction and understandings, that is, through discourses. Discourses are sets of physical, behavioural and cognitive practices that generate knowledge of bodies, experience, phenomena and subjectivities. In *The Birth of the Clinic*, Foucault (1976) describes how physical examination practices in the early medical clinics led to a way of seeing ('the gaze') that enabled physicians to develop an understanding of pathological anatomy, which in turn led to the development of a medical discourse about the body. Such a discourse gave the developing medical profession disciplinary power over the body by rendering it an object to be understood through surveillance. Similarly, in *Discipline and Punish*, Foucault (1991[1975]) explored the way in which the prison system developed through the Panopticon, Bentham's architectural design in which cells built around the periphery surround a central tower, from which all the cells and their inmates can be viewed:

> By the effect of backlighting, one can observe from the tower, standing out precisely against the light, the small captive shadows in the cells of the periphery. They are like so many cages, so many small theatres, in which each actor is alone, perfectly individualised and constantly visible. The panoptic mechanism arranges spatial unities that make it possible to see constantly and to recognise immediately... Visibility is a trap.
>
> (p. 200)

The arrangement of the cells ensures that those surveilled are hidden from each other: 'He is seen, but he does not see; he is the object of information, never a subject in communication' (Foucault 1991 [1975]: 200). The effect is 'to induce in the inmate a state of conscious and permanent visibility that assures the automatic functioning of power'. Individuals watch themselves even when they are not being watched. Foucault's analysis of power in and through the Panopticon has provided a possible analytical approach to the analysis of power relations in health surveillance and in health care in the community.

Armstrong (1983) has adopted Foucault's genealogical method to explore the development of the Dispensary, a place for the screening, diagnosis and treatment of individuals thought to have tuberculosis, which developed towards the end of the nineteenth century, providing a new form of health care within the community. The Dispensary was located within the community. Its function was identifying and monitoring disease and the spread of disease. It was thus concerned not just with the body as anatomical, with an emphasis on pathology, but with the body as a social entity. The body has social relationships, in a social as well as a physical environment. As Nettleton (1995) notes, 'as surveillance extended into the community, the emphasis began to shift from those who were ill to those who were potentially ill' (p. 236).

A Foucauldian analysis of aspects of care in the community has also been developed by Bloor and McIntosh (1990) in their analysis of health visiting. They argued that health visitors operated within discourses that define acceptable standards of child development, parenting and lifestyles. Working-class mothers regarded health visitors as being involved in social control, making judgements about homes and behaviour. Health visiting is thus seen as being involved in social as well as health surveillance. Health visitors adopt a 'therapeutic gaze' which, as Porter (1996) identifies, 'constitutes people as psycho-social beings and involves observation, interpretation and redefinition of their behaviour' (p. 68). Foucault (1982) used the term 'pastoral power' to refer to power directed towards people as individual subjects.

Nettleton (1995) has described studies that adopt Foucault's methodology as exploring 'the differential ways in which bodies are regulated, understood and constructed' (p. 233). She identifies a progressive movement towards the construction of the 'whole person' as the object of health care, exemplified through changing discourses in approaches to alcohol consumption (Bunton 1990), in psychiatry (Prior 1991), in dentistry (Nettleton 1992), in health education and through a change towards risk-orientated practice (Castel 1991). Similarly, May (1992b) has explored nursing's development of holistic models of care as contributing to the development of the disciplinary power of the nurse through therapeutic surveillance.

Professional knowledge, professional practice and 'objects' of care

Two aspects of a Foucauldian analysis are of particular importance to an analysis of professional care. One is the examination of changing ways of constructing professional knowledge and associated professional practices, and the second is the identification of the *objects* that are constructed through the changing discourses that constitute changing knowledge bases and professional practices. Nettleton (1992), in her analysis of dentistry, identified how practices that were used to gain information about populations came to be linked to dental techniques and practices used at an individual level, constructing the objects of dental study. Thus epidemiological data about teeth accompanied the dentist's focus on visual inspection of the mouth and teeth. The object of study was the mouth. Later, the professional knowledge base of dentistry came to include survey data about social circumstances, beliefs and their effects on dental care. Professional practice emphasised supportive and negotiating strategies in communications with patients in order to change behaviour. Nettleton sees the object of care as being reconstructed as a subjective, participating person. Prior (1991) similarly argued that when patient *behaviour* became the object of psychiatric study, the rationale for institutionalised care diminished since the professional gaze could not logically be restricted to behaviour within an institution. The focus of psychiatric concern became not just mental illness but mental health, and the arena of practice became the community rather than just the institution. Similar changes in the focus of professional practice and in discourses about professional knowledge can be seen in the *Health of the Nation*'s emphasis on improving collective health status and on using epidemiological data to assess need and target resources to those most at risk (DoH 1992a). Castel (1991) has argued that the target of medical care is now an individual's characteristics and behaviour that have been constructed as risk factors. As in dentistry, since it is the individual who is seen as responsible for these risk factors, professionals are involved in negotiating with the subjective, participating client.

Nettleton (1995) extends this analysis to the focus on needs assessment within the community as a result of the NHS and Community Care Act (1990). The new focus on needs assessment can be seen as part of the reconfiguration of disciplinary power that has evolved through the shift towards care in the community and the accompanying development of holistic models of care. Broadening professional knowledge to include an understanding of social factors and individual psychology has led to new 'objects' of practice (individual needs) and to new professional practices. Assessing needs using a holistic model involves professional alliances between professional disciplines as well as alliances with clients, carers and other agencies. Disciplinary power implicit in holistic care is constructed through the tentacles of community networks and alliances, but it is also dependent on inter-professional collaboration and collaboration with the subjective participating client.

Background to community care

Means and Smith (1994) have suggested their own brief genealogy of the concept of community care and the origins of 'the positive power' of the term. Their policy analysis identifies the economic imperatives that have underlined changes in policy. Community care was initially constructed as opposed to institutional care and referred to a shift away from hospital- to community-based provision for people with learning disabilities and mental health difficulties. Discussions about community care came to include care of the elderly not in expensive hospitals but in residential homes and increasingly in their own homes (and at their own expense), supported by domiciliary services. Alongside assumptions that care in the community was better than institutional care was the expectation that it was cheaper. Progressively, as Means and Smith (1994) identify, care in the community came to mean care 'by the community' (DHSS 1981: 3), that is, informal care provided mainly by unpaid family members, particularly women (Dalley 1988). The approach adopted by the 1989 White Paper *Caring for People* (DoH 1989), however, has led to the term being used 'to refer to the full spectrum of care and services received by certain groups' (Means and Smith 1994: 3). Means and Smith see 'the positive power' of the term as stemming from the idyllic connotations of the term 'community', with connotations of social harmony, integration and support. These are interesting connotations set alongside a Foucauldian disciplinary analysis. Whereas social harmony and integration may themselves involve surveillance, there is an implicit suggestion that it is the community that has constructed its own knowledge. Professionals and professional discourses are absent from the *idyll* of community care.

The key objectives of community care, as laid out by *Caring for People* (DoH 1989), concerned the empowerment of service users through promoting choice and independence for people in their own homes, a 'proper assessment of need', support for carers and improved accountability for the performance of service providers. Further mechanisms for ensuring that care in the community would be sensitive to the needs of users and carers included enabling the development of a range of independent providers of services alongside public services and developing effective care management practices. Although the responsibility for care management was given to social services departments, with care managers acting as purchasers of services from a variety of providers on behalf of users and their carers, effective care management involves considerable co-operation between professional agencies and diverse other providers as well as collaboration between providers, users and their carers.

Surveillance and resistance in assessment of need

A Foucauldian analysis would suggest that the reforms set out the mechanisms for extensive disciplinary power through a network of shared surveillance in order to enable the 'proper assessment of need'. Shared assessment, however, involves shared understanding and teamwork. Opie (1997), in a review of research concerning professional teamwork, identifies significant problems, including difficulties in inter-professional teamwork and professional resistance to user-centred discourses. She notes the difficulties as being:

> lack of interprofessional trust resulting in complicated power relations between professions; an overabundance of or, alternatively, an absence of conflict; lack of clear structures and directions; unclear goals; the dominance of particular discourses resulting in the exclusion of others; the existence of tensions between professional discourses resulting in potentially unsafe practices; lack of continuity of members; difficulty of definition of key terms; the production of client discussions which, far from addressing client goals, marginalise them and contribute to clients' disempowerment; and an absence of teams' examination of their processes. (p. 262)

Barker (1993), in a summary of Foucault's main hypotheses about power, notes that, for Foucault, 'there are no relations of power without resistances, and these resistances are formed precisely where power is being exercised' (p. 78). Bloor and McIntosh (1990) found resistance to health visiting surveillance in their study of 80 working-class Glasgow mothers. Mothers challenged the legitimacy of health visitors' surveillance by denigrating health visitors' knowledge and emphasising mothers' practical experience and skill. Mothers also failed to follow health visitors' advice and adopted strategies of avoidance and concealment. If power is everywhere, resistance is everywhere.

One of the main sites of resistance to shared professional surveillance through effective teamworking lies in the discursive practices of different professional groups, which serve to perpetuate differences rather than agreement between care workers. It is these differences between professional discourses that can contribute to ineffective teamwork and a failure to meet needs.

Professional education and professional discourses

Many of the difficulties associated with inter-professional work are seen as deriving from the isolation of initial education programmes that allow separate cultures to develop. Beattie (1995) adopts an anthropological metaphor and explores the persistence of 'tribalism' among health care professions. Whereas such tribalism can be seen as developing through the class divisions and gender barriers that shaped the development of medicine and nursing as professions, specialist and separate training has also accentuated and inscribed separate identities, values and discourses. Becker *et al.* (1961), Merton (1957) and Hughes (1956) explored, using different sociological approaches, the process of socialisation into the medical profession through a distinctive educational system. Atkinson (1977, 1981) identified the hierarchical structure of knowledge and accompanying social relationships that contributed to the development of segmented specialist areas of medical practice in a Scottish medical school.

Ellis' research (1993) into user participation in needs assessment gives clear examples of the effects of initial education on the preconceptions of professional workers, preconceptions that significantly inhibited the involvement of user and carer in needs assessment and care management. Hence these professional discourses resisted the user-centred discourses of community care. Ellis (1993) found, for example, that both occupational therapists and social workers in a research study tended to see impairment in terms of loss and bereavement. Social workers saw their role as helping people to come to terms with their loss and prioritised dealing with deep emotions rather than practical difficulties. Practitioners involved with people with learning disabilities and with services for deaf people, in contrast, 'sought to tackle structural and attitudinal barriers as well as support the individual. Indeed deaf people were regarded less as disabled people than as members of a minority linguistic and cultural group' (p. 13). Home care managers saw themselves as using a 'streetwise' common sense approach to identifying ways of helping people to do what they could not do for themselves. Ellis' research suggests that the perpetuation and reaffirmation of individual professional discourses may promote resistance to multiprofessional teamwork.

Ellis (1993) identified how different discourses concerning needs, particularly differences in user and professional discourses, led to differences in needs assessment. One local authority social service department analysed referrals for simple equipment and found that less than a quarter of the users received the equipment they themselves requested. Some received nothing; most received something different. Whereas this could be justified by acknowledging the role of expert assessment, it can also be viewed as illustrating different interpretations of need. Ellis notes many examples of practitioners' stereotyped and judgemental responses concerning clients. Whereas 'many home care assessors seemed to regard cleanliness as much as an indicator of good character as of general well being' (p. 14), a group of occupational therapists noted a preference for letting clients struggle. Professional moralistic assumptions included using ways of assessing to 'catch people out' and seeing clients as 'demanding', 'grabbing', 'fussy' and 'institutionalised'. 'Practitioners preferred users and carers to be grateful' (p. 22).

Professionals can thus be seen as resisting the discourse that emphasises co-operation and collaboration between health care providers. There is also evidence of resistance to involving clients in their own needs assessment and care management. Whereas ineffective teamwork can reduce the extensive nature of surveillance, ineffective teamwork and failure to 'see' the clients as part of the team can lead to ineffective care.

Ellis' (1993) research identified many examples in which professional assessments failed to meet users' definitions of need. One older woman whose lifestyle had been radically altered through her loss of sight had lost confidence in her ability to go out alone. Loss of confidence was exacerbated by the effect of loss of weight and ill-fitting clothes. 'All she really wanted was somebody to take her out every now and then, particularly shopping.' The social worker, however, 'believed the case constituted a hierarchy of losses in which the traumatic loss of a parent was the most fundamental and unresolved issue'. The social worker doubted the rehabilitation officer's identification of lack of social contact as being the main issue and doubted the efficacy of rehabilitation training, seeing the older woman as 'emotionally housebound' (p. 32). Ellis' account of her research indicates many instances in which health and social care practitioners could be seen as not meeting needs but as practising a form of surveillance whereby what they saw was constructed through their own professional discourses. These discourses are themselves constructed and constrained by practitioners' own lack of control over time and resources, leading to practices that 'are more consistently directed towards ensuring their own survival than advocating on behalf of users and carers' (p. 39). Ellis concludes that user-centred community care requires a shift in emphasis towards 'the politics of negotiation' acknowledging that definitions of need are contested. This view is echoed by Opie (1997), who stresses the importance of professionals critiquing their own discursive practices. Opie argues:

> for the team to move beyond its repetitious modes of interaction, the familiarity of which reinforces their value, requires an awareness of the different discourses spoken by the team and of the resulting representations of clients. (p. 276)

Opie is proposing that an awareness of discursive practices leads to the possibility of new discourses that do enable partnerships. Such awareness and the opportunity to reflect on analytic processes involved in team discussions require time and training, factors that are rarely available. Recalling Foucault's own arguments about resistance, however, professional practices are themselves effective forms of resistance to multiprofessional surveillance.

Nurses, discourses and multiprofessional teams

If Opie is right in that an ability to critique the discursive mode of production of models of practice and the objects of practice is a precursor to successful multidisciplinary teamwork, nurses' own education may in itself inhibit a conscious and reflexive analysis of competing, contradictory or shared discourses. Nurses traditionally play a subordinate role in health care teams, and the processes of disempowerment, explored in earlier chapters, are not changed by the rhetoric of collaborative teamwork. Melia (1987) found that student nurses learned a range of versions of the nature of nursing work with different expectations of the nurse's role. Students coped with conflicting expectations by conforming to expectations in each setting, with consequent limitations on students' confidence and assertiveness. Melia notes how nurses deal with internal tensions in relationships with other professions:

> when it comes to its dealings with other health care disciplines the group must be able to produce and rely upon a united front... the students learn not to expose the differences as they pass between segments during their training – instead they 'fit in' and 'move on'.
>
> (1987: 183)

Nursing can thus mask its differences through a spurious consensus and through oppressive domination by the majority. Oppressed professionals and nurses who are ignorant about the skills of other nurses are not likely to be constructive change agents. Thornton (1997) found community nurses to be unaware of other nurses' role. In her study of primary health care teams' perceptions of the needs of adults with learning disabilities living in the community, she found that 'one district nurse said she was ashamed to admit that she was not aware that community nurses were working with people with learning disabilities and a health visitor expressed surprise that the professional status of such nurses equalled her own' (p. 52).

Nurses' confidence in their own role in health care teams suffers through their lack of control over their work conditions and their lack of control over decision making. Kennedy and Grey (1997), in a study on causes of nurses' stress, report that whereas working in a team was a positive aspect of nurses' work, poor communication with other professionals, particularly doctors, was rated negatively. A case study reported in *Nursing Times* (1997), described a nurse's experience of being 'grilled by three managers' and a consultant who wanted to know why she had given a patient information about his heart condition, which had led to the patient refusing to co-operate with an exercise test. An attempt to work outside the dominant medical discourse had led to a loss of confidence and difficulty in working effectively. Nurses' lack of leadership experience and their limited involvement in multidisciplinary management roles do not suggest that nurses are likely to play a key role in promoting user involvement in needs assessment in community care, or that community care teams will enable nurses to enhance their status and role as practitioners.

Nevertheless, nurses' learned capacity to 'fit in' and 'move on' irrespective of the dominant discourse can make them essential, albeit submissive, members of the team. Nurses' tolerance of different rituals and practices within different areas of nursing practice may make tolerance of other professionals' ways of seeing relatively unproblematic. Despite the professionalising discourses developed through nursing theories and nursing models, many nurses have continued to practise with a practical, common sense orientation to their work, leaving lay biases and prejudices relatively untouched by analytical exploration of the human condition. Ellis (1993) found that a community nurse rejected the view that assessment of need required professional expertise. The nurse felt that, to equalise relations between practitioner and user, practitioners should present themselves as human and fallible rather than professional and in control. Nurses' respect for what Benner (1984) described as intuition may in itself allow individual nurses to respond easily to clients' own definitions of need. Furthermore, nursing's traditionally strong emphasis on individualised, patient-focused care can be seen as accommodating the discourse of user involvement without difficulty, although nurses' care orientation can be seen by service users as promoting dependency rather than participatory assessment of need. Porter (1996), however, has argued that 'clients of "New Nursing" have gained considerably more in terms of their own knowledge and autonomy than they have lost in terms of nurses' knowledge of them' (p. 76).

Changing discourses in nursing practice in the community

There is some evidence to suggest that nurses are responding creatively to care in the community. Far from allowing competing professional discourses to inhibit the development of client-centred teamwork, nurses are developing new ways of working in the community. Watkins and Wilson (1997) have described a public health nursing project in Stockport whereby health visitors drew on their experience with community health needs assessment and health promotion to work with other agencies in community development work. The underlying principles of the work are co-ordination, co-operation, collaboration, community action and community development. The case for such an approach is that 'creating a community which can address its own problems and where people work together, establishes more effective partnerships with authority' (p. 44). In Foucauldian terms, this could be seen as public health nursing as panoptic surveillance. The Stockport project involves the development of new discourses, new practices and new objects of study (the community).

Ness and Ryrie (1997) describe a client-orientated and community-based service for people with severe mental health problems in Lambeth in which nurses have organised themselves into teams providing assessment and treatment, case management and outreach work, liaising successfully with each other and with other services. Nurses successfully combine what the authors describe as:

> a clinical and co-ordinator approach to case management. Acting as co-ordinator the nurse links up with a range of other services as diverse as housing, leisure, employment, legal and financial. He or she also ensures that the client has adequate access to primary care and other health and social services. (p. 39)

The successful negotiation of change has been accompanied by staff development and training, largely through the Thorn Nurse Training Programme, which has enabled practitioners to reflect on discourses underpinning mental health care and to begin to work with changing models of practice incorporating both psychosocial interventions and an increased emphasis on community outreach work. The 'object' of care is certainly seen as a social being. Similarly, McMillan (1997) reports on the Drayton Park crisis centre for women, winner of the 1996 Sainsbury Mental Health award, which provides a community-based service for women, staffed by women. Not all the staff are nurses, and Shirley McNicholas, responsible for developing the project, stresses the importance of women staff drawing on their own experience as women to inform their practice. The significance of this approach lies in the recognition of the role that personal as opposed to professional discourses can play in community care. Some mental health practitioners are exploring new approaches to mental health care, based on the view that clients have a central role to play in their own recovery. Baker (1997), for example, offers four practical ways to forge alliances with users. These are:

> redefining relationship with users. Work with voice hearers and survivor groups can acknowledge the validity of clients' understandings and explanations of their problems;
>
> developing a new language. The term 'voice hearer', for example, validates the client's understanding through using clients own words for the experience;
>
> social action as a way to develop partnerships. 'Community development or social action... assumes that the knowledge, experience and skills of groups of people can be harnessed to bring about constructive change based on their own agendas' (p. 42);
>
> the importance of service users as educators. Service users have been involved in the education of mental health workers.

All these strategies suggest a willingness on the part of mental health nurses to engage in reflective analysis of their own and others' explanatory discourses. Clients' understandings and explanations are given validity alongside professional knowledge. Changing discourses about knowledge accompany changing practice, involving alliances both with community groups and with service users themselves. The object of care is a subjective participating client, living in a social world (a community). If such changes are widespread, mental health nursing could have an impact on changing discourses in community care.

These examples of inter-professional teamwork and client partnerships could be seen as part of a reconfiguration of disciplinary power facilitated by nurses' newly developed practices of surveillance in the community. Such changes in practice do suggest that nurses can play a role in overcoming the resistance to collaborative user-centred community care. Through facilitating collaborative user-centred community care, nurses may have a positive role to play in ensuring that individual needs are met and managed in an enabling manner. Foucault's work, however, suggests that collaborative community care may equally well become an effective and possibly repressive means of panoptic surveillance. Porter (1996) has criticised Foucault's contention that power is everywhere as leading to an inability to distinguish between different instances of surveillance and to what he termed 'praxical paralysis', that is, an inability to seek change. This is an important point, for if an analysis of power does not enable nurses to distinguish between repressive and positive power, empowering nursing practice is unobtainable and unimaginable. If nursing action is ultimately surveillance, participative and enabling practice is futile. Paradoxically, resisting the discourses of teamwork in community care would leave users more space for their own resistance strategies.

However, it is not clear that Foucault's pervasive power is necessarily repressive. In existing through relationships, interaction, understandings, through discourses that generate knowledge of bodies, individuals and needs, discursive power may promote health. If the relationships, interactions and understandings are shaped and reshaped through both resistance and surveillance, professional and client participation and exchange may result. Foucault (1980) notes that power 'doesn't only weigh on us a force that says no, but it traverses and produces things, it induces pleasure, forms knowledge, produces discourse' (p. 119). Teamwork in community care could be described similarly, as the force that says no, or as the productive force that induces pleasure, forms knowledge and produces new practices and objects of care. Using Foucault's analyses to recognise the potential for panoptic community surveillance can help to reveal the importance of professionals critiquing their own discursive practice while they develop new models of interprofessional practice.

PART IV

Relationships with clients

9 Disempowerment, empowerment and older people

Drew Thomas

Introduction

This chapter is concerned with the relative powerlessness of a group of people who are defined solely by their age. However, viewing those (for the sake of argument) over the age of 65 as a separate and special case for investigation could be seen as disempowering in itself. By doing this, older people are being grouped together, ghettoised, seen as different from the rest of the population. Yet failing to identify older people as singularly disadvantaged in this society is to run the risk of ignoring the processes and effects of the way in which a large section of our population is, simply because of their chronological age, denied full participation in the decision making that affects their lives.

This chapter seeks to examine the causes and effects of older peoples' relative powerlessness in our society. First, an overall view of the social processes that disempower older people is examined; then the unequal nature of their interaction with the health care professions will be explored. The second part of the chapter offers a critical account of social policy and health care practices that have attempted to overcome the power differential that exists between older users of the health services and those who manage and implement those services. It looks at the NHS and Community Care Act 1990's claim to empower service users and examines strategies intended to empower elderly people in their encounters with nursing practice.

The processes of disempowerment

This chapter takes as its starting point the idea that the nature of being old in contemporary society is largely the result of social factors. This idea challenges what could be seen as the common sense view that the experience of old age is determined by the biological processes of ageing. The notion of old age being 'socially constructed' requires further explanation.

To describe an aspect of our social life as socially constructed is to argue that it is as it is because of the social forces that create it. It may be easier to see the position of women in society as being socially constructed than it is to view the experience of old age as a social construction. Many women find themselves fulfilling two major roles: one as a home maker, the other as a wage earner. Women thus have a 'dual role' involving a range of responsibilities (Abbott and Wallace 1990: 146). This has not always been the case but has been created by the social pressures of changing patterns of employment and by the persistence of ideas about women's 'natural' roles as housewives and mothers. It can be argued that it is not inevitable for women to experience the double burden of unpaid domestic labour and paid employment outside the home – it does not have to be like this. Men could take an equal responsibility for housework, and workplace nurseries could become the norm, which would alter women's experience of both work and home life.

In contrast to this example of women's socially constructed roles, as we grow older our circumstances clearly do change because we are subject to a biological process, namely ageing. Biologists can accurately describe, and to an extent explain, our decline in physical functioning as we grow older. Similarly, psychologists can demonstrate changes, usually (but not always) in terms of the decline of our cognitive functions. Furthermore, we all know that these things happen – the evidence is all around us and within ourselves. However, the biological analysis is not, on its own, sufficient to explain the actual experience of old age. Old age is not necessarily seen as a period of retirement and economic inactivity in all cultures. Overall, two mutually reinforcing mechanisms can be identified as constructing the experience of old age: first, the economic position of elderly people in this society, and second, ageism, which is the stereotyping of, and resultant prejudice and discrimination against, older people.

Retirement makes older people economically dependent upon the rest of society and more likely to be in poverty than other groups. As Walker (1990) points out, however, old age is not the cause of poverty; social policies and economic forces have combined to create this situation. Retirement at a specific age is a clear, although arbitrary, mark of the end of an individual's economically active life. It is purely a social construct and one which has a profound effect on how people experience old age. Fennell *et al.* (1988) argue that one must look at changing family structures and the way in which families and the state (and, they could have added, the voluntary sector) provide support, particularly for frail older people, to gain a fuller picture of the ways in which the economic dependency of older people is socially constructed. Such factors have nothing to do with the biological processes of ageing but are governed by economic circumstances and social policy decisions.

Ageism is linked to the economic position of older people in so far as retirement is both a cause and an effect of the low expectations of the contribution that elderly people can make to society. Johnson and Bytheway (1993) see ageism, as applied to older people, not only as having 'institutional' effects such as compulsory retirement. They also describe 'interpersonal' effects in the way in which elderly people are regarded. At the root of this is the presumption that, following a purely biological model of decline, to be old is to be inferior to, and therefore separate and different from, the general population. This can be used to legitimate a denial of 'resources and opportunities' that are available to the rest of the population (Bytheway and Johnson 1990: 36). This is legitimated by retirement, which provides an institutional expression of economic dependence and separation from 'mainstream' society.

It is the social construction of old age that leads to the disempowerment of elderly people. While the biological facts of physical decline cannot be denied, such decline does not in itself result in the disempowerment of old people (Johnson 1991, Johnson and Bytheway 1993). Disempowerment is a result of the structuring of social roles of older people. Older people are marginalised from the rest of society by what Townsend (1986) describes as the 'restriction of domestic and community roles'. This marginalisation leads to older people being given, and taking, a passive role in relation to the formation of social policies that often affect them greatly (Biggs 1993). The very presentation of social policies that address the fact that there are increasing numbers of older people in the population tends to do so in terms of older people being a problem and a burden upon the rest of society (Fennell *et al.*

1988). An article in the *Guardian*, for example, reporting on the effects of demographic changes, did so under the headline 'Time running out to avert elderly crisis'. Jones (1994) argues that expressing policy issues in such a way influences the construction of dependency of older people through assuming, incorrectly, that the majority of older people are dependent in the physical sense while at the same time reinforcing the socially constructed economic dependency of older people who are no longer members of the workforce. Furthermore, being viewed as dependent is to be labelled as deviant, as a group who do not deserve to enjoy the full benefits of society (Johnson 1990). Hence older people become further disempowered.

The line of argument followed in this chapter so far could be criticised for seeming to assume tacitly that all those over the age of 65 years form a homogenous group who will experience the disempowerment that is associated with old age in the same way and to the same degree. However, individuals and groups are disempowered because of gender, disability, class, race and sexuality as well as age (Mitchell 1989). The ageism and economic disadvantage experienced by older people in our society are clearly exacerbated by the disadvantage resulting from belonging to a lower socio-economic group. Similarly, it is exacerbated for older members of minority ethnic groups by racism and for older women by sexism (Fennell *et al.* 1988). There appears to be very little work on the experience of older lesbians and gay men, although McDougal (1993) suggests that older gay men and lesbians have developed coping social and psychological mechanisms that result in them entering old age with advantages over their heterosexual counterparts. However, oppression on grounds of age encompasses all groups in society (Biggs 1993). While the experience of an older, white middle-class man can be expected to be very different from that of an older, black working-class woman, they will both be disempowered because of their chronological age, irrespective of the disempowerment that results from other social divisions. To concentrate on the disadvantage experienced by people as they grow older is not to minimise or ignore the effects of disadvantages that result from other social divisions; it is to examine a unique form of oppression that affects people simply because of their age.

Older people and health services

The relationship between the lay person of any age and the health professional is an unequal one, and this inequality is inherently disempowering (Malin and Teasdale 1991, Stevenson and Parsloe 1993). The inequity of the relationship is based not just upon the superior knowledge of health and illness that a professional is perceived to possess, but also on the way in which that knowledge is used to limit patients' choices, to control behaviour, particularly in institutional settings, and even to define who is, and who is not, a patient and therefore in need of treatment (Hugman 1991). Changing patterns of illness throughout life mean that, as we grow older, we are more likely to come into contact with the health services. Older people are major users of health care and, as a group, account for more than half of the NHS budget (Jones 1994). Those over the age of 75 years are about twice as likely to suffer from chronic ill health than are the population as a whole and around three times more likely to have an acute episode of illness (Office of Health Economics 1995). Hence, older people not only suffer the oppression that arises from living in an ageist society, but are also more likely than the general population to suffer from the disempowerment that results from being a lay service user in contact with a professional group.

This situation is compounded when it is seen that the administration and delivery of health services are demonstrably ageist. Henwood (1993) points out that debates about the allocation of limited health care resources are presented in terms of an intergenerational conflict, which reflects the idea of older people being a 'burden' on 'the rest' of society. The result is a chronically under-resourced service, particularly for those who need services on a long-term basis, in contrast to the high profile of acute and high-tech health care. A clear example of the effect of this is what Henwood (1992) describes as the policy 'by default' (p. 9) of effectively moving the care provision of older people, whose level of impairment means that they need long-term nursing care, out of the NHS and into the private sector. The provision of such care is means tested, and many people have to pay. Hence the financial 'burden' of providing this care is relieved to an extent, and the view of the NHS as an acute service, which does not have a duty of care towards older people who cannot be cured, is reinforced.

Specific aspects of the operation of health services can be seen to be discriminatory against older people. Henwood (1993) cites the lack of cervical screening by the NHS for women over the age of 65 and the complete absence of screening for osteoporosis as examples of this. There is no medical reason to have an age limit for screening for cervical cancer (Henwood 1993). Osteoporosis, primarily a disease of older women, reduces bone density and dramatically increases the probability of sustaining serious fractures. The mortality following a fractured hip is 15–20 per cent, and of those who survive, a further 20 per cent fail to make a full functional recovery (Larsson *et al.* 1995). Such operational effects of the ageist assumptions upon which such an unequal allocation of resources are based can be seen in terms of what Lukes (1974) describes as the second face of power. Ageist assumptions have set the health policy agenda that allows for the oppression of a group who are already economically disadvantaged. Lukes' formulation sees the exercise of power in terms of controlling the agenda of decision making so that potential conflict is stifled. This results in policies that discriminate against older people rather than policies that allow older people to take more control of their lives and to be active in decision making processes that affect them. In the all-pervading nature of ageism can also be seen the operation of Lukes' third face of power, in which 'the bias of the system is not sustained simply by a series of individually chosen acts, but also, most importantly, by the socially structured and culturally patterned behaviour of groups' (Lukes 1974: 13). This leads to both decisions and non-decisions being seen as 'common sense', with no rational alternative, so dominant is the discourse of ageism.

Any episode of illness involving a degree of dependency on others can result in a loss of power to control events. Becoming a hospital patient, at whatever age, involves a certain loss of autonomy (Bond and Bond 1994), and there are particular difficulties for older people entering hospital. Brown and Furstenberg (1992) identify a tendency by staff to assume the level of physical and mental competence that they observe when the older person is acutely ill to be their normal level of functioning. Underlying this are ageist stereotypes that affect all their interactions with the patient and can lead to an underestimation of an individual's capabilities. This exacerbates the passivity and loss of control and choice that all patients experience in hospital. Such attitudes can work against the model of rehabilitative care that an older person may require following an acute illness.

People who are made vulnerable by a health crisis and resulting hospitalisation are not in a strong position to exercise choice. However, Hoyes *et al.* (1993) point out that this is often what older people are required to do when asked to make decisions on such a crucial issue as whether they feel able to return to their own home on discharge from hospital, or whether they should enter a nursing or residential home. Despite recent reforms to the provision of community care, there remains evidence that direct power is exerted, particularly by medical staff, to move people, usually older people, who are seen as 'bed blockers', out of the acute hospital sector once an immediate health crisis has been stabilised (Marks 1994). This is possible because of the ability of the medical profession to control the discourse concerning the purpose of hospitals and the boundaries of the practice of medicine. It is done by presenting the hospital sector as purely one of the short-term management of acute illness and the practice of medicine as being purely directed towards effecting a cure. People who have chronic disabilities or are in need of long-term rehabilitation are seen as not responding to treatment by doctors and, by association, not deserving of hospital care (Age Concern England 1993). In this way, it is possible for the NHS to withdraw from the provision of long-term nursing care. It also makes it possible for medical and other hospital staff to exert pressure to achieve an early discharge of an older person from hospital. The older patient is often perceived as being passive in the process of choosing between options for long-term care, the tendency being for an individual's relatives or carers to make choices on their behalf, thus compounding their disempowerment (Brown and Furstenberg 1992). As a result, older people generally do not go into residential care; instead they are 'put there by someone else' (Booth 1993: 160).

The disempowerment of many older people who live in residential or nursing homes can be immense, although it should be noted that only just over 3 per cent of those over 65 years of age and 6 per cent of those over 75 live in such settings (Office of Health Economics 1995). The roots of the disempowerment that older people experience in such institutions can be found within the self-fulfilling assumption identified by Booth (1993); the very fact that they are in need of the care that the home provides demonstrates that they are unable to make choices and manage their own lives. He goes on to describe the process of assimilation of the residents into the value structure of the home whereby they become passive recipients of care. This lack of a voice for such older people can be seen as being the result of the exercise of all three faces of power as identified by Lukes (1974).

The first dimension of power – direct, overt decision making – can be seen in the deprivation of choice, for example of where to sit or when to get up, that characterises the regimes in some nursing and residential homes (Redfern 1991).

The second face of power – the setting of the agenda that determines the environment in which the residents live – can be used very effectively in institutional settings and can particularly be seen if the routine of the home is focused upon the smooth running of the institution rather than the individual needs of the residents. It becomes 'very difficult to complain if you do not perceive yourself as having any choice' (Booth 1993: 162).

Finally, and arguably the most effective use of power by any institution, is the ability to get residents to identify with the processes and procedures of that institution and to see them as being in their interests even when, viewed from outside, the interests of the institution and those of the residents are very different and may well be in opposition to each other. Booth (1993) provides an insight into this when he suggests that, when studying residents' attitudes, the expressions of satisfaction with their circumstances that such research commonly reveals cannot safely be taken to be a genuine reflection of their feelings. This may be, as Redfern (1991) suggests, because residents fear reprisals if they complain, or simply because they cannot see any alternative to their current situation. As Booth (1993) points out, such residents are very isolated in their home and are not in a position to compare their situation with that of others.

Empowering older people – social policy

The literature identifies two broad aspects of empowerment. First is the 'micro' approach, which concentrates on the relationship between the professional and client, as characterised by Malin and Teasdale (1991). They argue that, in order to address the power differential between nurse and patient, the nurse must become the patients' partner, placing his or her expertise at their disposal, enabling them to make independent choices about their health care. The second, 'macro', approach can be seen as more radical in that, while it encompasses the micro position, it goes further by addressing the root causes of the powerlessness that affects clients. For Gibson (1991), while empowering patients means that nurses must develop relationships that will enable patients to take responsibility for their own care, the nurse must, as part of this process, also consider the wider social factors that may affect health. This will include such social divisions as age and class and may also involve challenging the system of health care delivery.

This section will examine this final aspect of empowerment by concentrating on the implications of the NHS and Community Care Act 1990 for the relationship between older people as users of services and the organisations and professionals who provide them. The next section will explore both the micro level of empowerment at the individual level and the broader issues of what Hughes (1995) describes as anti-ageist practice.

The National Health Service and Community Care Act 1990 attempts to address government concern at the inflexibility and lack of user choice in the provision of community care (Hughes 1995). The Act affects older people more than any other single group, in that older people are more likely to need support if they are to continue living in their own homes. Hughes (1995) summarises the government's agenda as aiming to address, first, the lack of alternatives to residential and nursing home placement for older people who need some sort of social or nursing support, and second, the rising cost of these options as the number of older people increases. In addition, the situation was seen as an opportunity to introduce market principles into the provision of community care and to increase the roles of both the private and voluntary sectors.

The Act aims to increase the involvement of the users of community services by their direct involvement in the assessment process by which an individual's needs are established. Of primary importance in this process is that the assessment is 'needs led' and not based on the level of service provision that is available or on the perceived eligibility of an individual to receive assistance. Following on from assessment, an individualised package of care will be developed to meet the identified needs (with monitoring of those needs that cannot be met because of financial restrictions or the unavailability of a particular service). Finally, the NHS and Community Care Act 1990 gives responsibility to local authorities to become purchasers of care from private or voluntary agencies, while at the same time reducing their roles as direct providers of services (Hughes 1995). Of particular interest in the context of this chapter is the way in which the Act affects the relationship between the older person and the providers of the services that they require, in other words, how older people operate as consumers in the market place of care and how this affects their power to influence decisions that relate to them.

The Department of Health/Social Services Inspectorate (1991) clearly identified one of the rationales for the new legislation as the 'empowerment of users and carers'. Users of community services are seen as consumers who make choices in a market place that provides a variety of care options, such as domiciliary support or respite care, provided by a variety of agencies that may be run by the private or voluntary sectors, or by the NHS or social services departments. The effect that the NHS and Community Care Act 1990 has in addressing the relative powerlessness of older people depends first upon what is meant by 'empowerment' and second upon the degree of influence that older people have over the nature and quality of the services that they need, and upon the level of choice between service providers.

Hoyes *et al.* (1993) and Taylor *et al.* (1992) see empowerment in relation to an organisation as being on a continuum, with different levels of user empowerment based upon the degree of influence over decisions. At one end of the continuum, where users have high levels of involvement, users have the authority to take decisions, or the authority to take selected decisions. A lower level of involvement occurs when users are able to influence decisions and/or users' views are sought before decisions are finalised. If decisions are publicised and explained before implementation, and information is given about the decisions made, the degree of empowerment is low. This formulation is essentially one of defining degrees of empowerment at the micro level. To judge the National Health Service and Community Care Act 1990 on this basis seems reasonable, in that the intention of the Act was never to pursue a vision of empowerment that encouraged challenges to the wider social processes that led to the disempowerment of any group. However, even on this limited basis, criticisms can be levelled at the operations of the Act for the extent of empowerment that it allows. Hoyes *et al.* (1993) point out that there is in fact a very limited choice of agencies that are in a position to deliver the required services and that the Act does not give consumers any direct purchasing power themselves. It is for this reason that Means *et al.* (1994) describe the welfare provision of the Act as operating as a 'quasi market', one in which the consumers' choices are 'mediated' by a care manager. This role of purchaser is taken by local authorities, which hold a limited budget and which are also, as Stevenson and Parsloe (1993) point out, ultimately responsible for the assessment of an individual's needs. However, Taylor *et al.* (1992) argue that such a quasi market system for the delivery of community services can potentially lead to greater user empowerment provided that there is adequate funding for services and that professionals consciously foster relationships with clients that are focused on user empowerment. This is also stressed by Hughes (1995), who argues that, within a market of care, it is possible for professionals to adopt an approach that focuses on the needs of clients rather than on those of the organisation. While this could be seen as empowering in a limited sense, it must be noted that the content of the assessment and the validity of the needs are determined by the assessor, in what can be seen as an exercise in agenda setting by professionals. Taylor *et al.* (1992) also make the point that empowerment in a market place would be greatly enhanced by incorporating into the system of care delivery the principle of consumer rights as opposed to needs. In other words, the consumer would not only have choice (at least theoretically) between different service providers, and be able to influence the nature of the provision, but would also be guaranteed rights to specific services, to decent housing, to freedom from discrimination and poverty.

Such an approach is a significant move away from assessing the level of individual empowerment provided for by the legislation. When a more macro perspective is adopted, the Act is found to be lacking. Empowerment through consumer choice is essentially a micro approach. It does not allow for challenges to the principle

- for their social and cultural histories.

Older people should have knowledge:

- about their conditions and prospects
- about ways of improving their situation
- about who is ultimately responsible for their care.

These are echoed in the principles of empowerment outlined by Booth (1993: 166), which see the empowerment of older people as needing to be 'proactive' in that care should be focused on an individual's capabilities rather than disabilities; it should be 'enabling' in that a person's abilities are encouraged to be used to constructive and fulfilling ends; and finally it should foster the 'independence' of older people, so that they have the maximum control over their own life. Hughes (1995) advocates the adoption of an 'anti-ageist practice' (p. 47), which includes the essence of Booth's principles but appears to take these ideas further with the use of the concept of normalisation to counteract the marginalising effects of ageism. This is the 'making available whatever is necessary to enable old people to carry on living in the same way, with the same or better quality of life as other people in society' (p. 47). In one respect, it is possible to see this in terms of a macro approach to empowerment in that, to achieve normalisation for older people, it would be necessary to challenge the institutions and ideologies of an ageist society. Hughes, however, in discussing the practicalities of operating by anti-ageist principles, gives further insights that demonstrate how this idea can be empowering on an individual level. She suggests the importance of, while taking account of the older people's views, not being limited by their own low expectations, which are the result of ageism. This could be seen as an example of recognising the operation of the third face of power (Lukes 1974). While the older person accepts the effects of living in an ageist society as the norm, the nurse can challenge those assumptions with the aim of improving clients' quality of life or the level of services that they receive. This demands a very positive attitude from the nurse, who needs to look for opportunities rather than barriers. This could be as simple as exploring the possibility of finding a voluntary organisation that could take older persons, who had assumed themselves to be housebound, shopping.

The picture can become complicated when nurses encounter patients who do not wish to be empowered. Salvage (1992) points out that not all patients want to be in partnership with a nurse, nor do they all wish to have control over decisions that affect them. She suggests that, in some circumstances, dependence on the nurse can have therapeutic benefits for the patient. Malin and Teasdale (1991) argue that there are occasions when giving patients all the relevant information to enable them to make an informed choice would simply heighten their anxiety without in any way empowering them. Using the ideas of Hughes (1995) to combat the low expectations of some older people and the dependency that results from ageism could be helpful here. However, on an individual level, it is possible to see ethical difficulties in persistently challenging a frail older person's wish for a degree of dependency, even if, in an ideal world, it could be seen as the unwanted product of an ageist society.

There is a tacit assumption in much that is written about advocacy and empowerment in relation to older people that the clients concerned are able to express their wishes. This is clearly not always the case. Hillan (1993), when considering older people with dementing illnesses, defends paternalism as a valid and benign principle upon which to base nursing care in circumstances in which the autonomy of the patient is judged to be an unrealistic goal. Stevenson and Parsloe (1993) come to similar conclusions when considering both health and social care in a community setting. They are concerned about the need to protect some clients from harm, but are also concerned that such ideas are not easily compatible with the principle of empowering patients. However, they point out that it is not a stark choice between empowerment and protection in that, while clients may have lost autonomy in some areas of their life, this may not be so for all areas. They suggest working out the relative importance of different activities in a client's life so that efforts can be concentrated towards maintaining autonomy in those areas which are most important to the client. As professional carers, nurses have to make difficult decisions that involve balancing clients' autonomy and their need for protection, but in doing so it is essential that the focus is on the client. Crucially, as Stevenson and Parsloe (1993) stress, in planning care with clients, all care workers must be aware of the effects of professional power and 'be aware of excessive anxiety and over-protectiveness in themselves or of the hidden satisfaction which they derive from the benign exercise of power' (p. 21).

A potentially quite radical contribution to approaching such situations is made by Gwilliam and Gilliard (1996), who apply the social model of disability to the environment in which people with dementia live and receive care, whether at home or in an institution. They argue that the extent to which the cognitive impairments caused by dementia are disabling depends upon the social environment in which the person with dementia lives. Advocating a multidisciplinary approach, they see it as the responsibility of professional carers to find ways in which 'an individual's surroundings can be simplified to a manageable level, [so that] an enabling environment can be created' (p. 15). Such an approach seems to represent a synthesis of the principles of empowerment, and in some cases the need for protection, of frail older people.

In view of the difficulties that older people face in relation to the operations of the NHS, and more broadly as consumers in the quasi market place created by the NHS and Community Care Act 1990, advocacy appears to be a fruitful avenue for the nurse to explore. Wertheimer (1993) and Phillipson (1993) both see advocacy as being particularly useful at times when older people are especially vulnerable, such as when they are ill and yet have to make decisions about treatment, when considering moving into residential care, and when arranging their discharge from hospital. In addition, advocacy provides a voice for the wishes of the older person faced with the power of professionals or institutions. Phillipson also sees that an advocacy service could seek to 'highlight injustices in old age' (p. 182). This is perceiving advocacy as empowering to older people in a more macro sense of extending their power to influence policy decisions and challenge ageism.

More commonly, advocacy is seen as a way of increasing client participation in choices about treatment or service provision. However, it does raise problems in its implementation. There is an argument, put clearly by the UKCC, that the nurse should when appropriate 'plead the cause of another', which involves the nurse making decisions 'in the best interests' of a patient who is unable to make informed choices him or herself (UKCC 1989b: 12) A number of authors have concluded that, with reservations, the nurse can act as an advocate for a patient (Ellis 1992, Graham 1992). All these sources acknowledge that there are some barriers to the nurse becoming a successful advocate. Specifically, they highlight the lack of experience and preparation that many nurses have for the role and the potential for conflict with other sections of the organisation for which the nurse works. Graham (1992) points out that such a conflict could arise if the nurse were pressing for more resources on behalf of a client. An example of this would be an issue such as a reduction in the provision of incontinence pads for users living in the community, where an aspect of resource allocation directly affects the service offered to a specific client or group. Inter-professional conflict can arise if, for example, advocacy involves a challenge to a doctor's decision about the 'best interests' of a patient. Penn (1994) illustrates this in the context of palliative care, in which nurses often develop close relationships with patients that enable them to gain insight into the patients' wishes. If these wishes run counter to the medical view of their best interests and the patients are too unwell to challenge the doctor themselves, the nurse may feel able to plead their case, although this will involve conflict with a colleague.

While these authors do not see these difficulties as insurmountable, what seems to be ignored is the power differential between the nurse and the patient, and how this is to be overcome if the nurse is to act in the patient's 'best interests'. Allmark and Klarzynski (1992) point out the vital distinction between pleading patients' causes and acting in their best interests. The former is true advocacy and may involve advocates putting a case that they themselves do not see as being in the patient's best interest. On the other hand, determining a patient's best interests may involve a professional nursing judgement with which the patient does not agree. For example, it might be a nurse's view that an older person is at significant physical risk if remaining in his or her own home, even with the maximum support available, and that the best option would be to go into residential care. If the client is not in agreement, he or she would need an independent advocate to put the case if unable to do so personally.

Wertheimer (1993) acknowledges that, in the short term, professionals can act as advocates, but she argues this is far from ideal and that conflicts of interest are bound to interfere with the role. Areas that seem potentially most likely to result in such conflicts would seem to be around issues of the restriction of choice or options in packages of care, access to information and the allocation of resources. Wertheimer (1993) suggests both that long-term partnerships should be fostered between advocates and older clients, and that short-term or 'crisis advocacy' (p. 42) should be available to support people through a specific episode. The longest running advocacy schemes for older people in Britain have only been in existence for a few years. They are all local voluntary schemes, and many areas of the country do not have one. This is clearly a problem for elderly people who require support when faced with the need to increase their level of participation in decision making processes that affect them. What may be a potentially greater problem in the long term may be, as both Wertheimer (1993) and Phillipson (1993) point out, a reluctance on the part of professionals and institutions to accept the role of an advocacy service. If it is not the role of the nurse to be a true advocate, it may be the nurses' role to ensure that they themselves, their colleagues and the organisation for which they work are receptive to their older clients' advocates.

Conclusion

The processes of the disempowerment of older people are complex, but the effects are clear. The stigma attached to old age allows older people to be marginalised from society and from its decision making processes in general, and in particular prevents them wielding any influence over health and social services. This is despite the fact that, as a group, older people are the heaviest users of those services. Although it pays lip service to the empowerment of clients, the NHS and Community Care Act 1990 does not address these fundamental inequities that are firmly rooted in ageism. Older people, often when at their most vulnerable, are frequently denied a choice between options and a voice within the service organisation, which would be unthinkable for a younger person.

The challenge for nurses lies in combating this disempowerment not only as it affects the lives of individual clients, but also in terms of the ageism that is endemic in society and which allows the oppression of older people to persist. This involves adopting such generalist approaches as Hughes' (1995) 'anti-ageist practice' and also ensuring that the focus of any involvement must always be on the needs of the client, even if that means that empowerment is not to be the ultimate goal (Stevenson and Parsloe 1993).

10 User empowerment within mental health nursing

Anthony Fraher and Michel Limpinnian

Introduction

This chapter explores issues surrounding user empowerment in mental health care settings, with particular reference to policy issues, to users' role in education and to the relationship between users and mental health nurses.

Origin and development of user empowerment: policy changes

The Mental Health Act 1959 began to address the empowerment of users, recognising the principle of voluntary admission and the right of appeal against continued detention for those of non-voluntary status. The 1983 Act gave right of appeal to the Mental Health Review Tribunal. In 1997 the Department of Health published additional requirements that demonstrate commitment to enhancing user empowerment in a practical way (DoH 1997b). Professionals directly involved in the care of those with mental health needs must supply detailed information about statutory mental health services, advocacy schemes and support groups in the users' locality. Professionals need to show that they are responding to users' rights by consulting them about proposed and alternative treatments and potential risks before gaining consent. Policy changes concerning care in the community have also emphasised empowering users and carers. The NHS and Community Care Act 1990 reflected a fundamental shift away from service-centred care towards a needs-led approach in which professionals are required to consult and develop partnerships with users and their carers when assessing needs. The Carers (Recognition and Services) Act 1995 requires professionals to take account of carers' views during the assessment process.

Beresford (1993) argues that dissatisfaction with paternalistic welfare provision throughout the post-war years allowed welfare service users' views to begin to influence political and policy agendas. Service users highlighted the fact that government policies did not address their needs. Groups representing users of mental health services prior to the 1980s, such as the Mental Patients' Union and the Campaign Against Psychiatric Oppression, shunned involvement in statutory services through lack of trust (Hopton 1995). Groups such as Survivors Speak Out, Psychiatric Survivor Movement and the United Kingdom Advocacy Network began to develop a more effective approach during the 1980s. Such groups focused on deficiencies in existing services and on the need for user involvement. However, it would be rash to conclude that it was the pressure of radical user groups alone that raised the importance of user empowerment within mental health policy. The prevailing political climate of the 1980s and early 1990s allowed New Right ideology to influence all aspects of the welfare state. New Right ideology emphasised minimal state intervention in individuals' lives and reliance on the free market as the most efficient means of distributing services, including welfare services. Market mechanisms can be seen as giving back consumer power to the individual. The role of user involvement in policy decision making was acknowledged. MIND (1992) argue, however, that users of the psychiatric services who have found a voice and a new sense of control over their lives often express the view that this was won in spite of, rather than through, mental health service provision. Indeed, not all recent policy changes can be seen as being in users' interests. Public alarm about safety has prompted the establishment of supervision registers, which have been severely criticised by user groups such as the Psychiatric Survivor Movement for creating a climate of disempowerment for the mentally ill. Government response, therefore, appears contradictory.

The nature of empowerment: exploring the issues

Gibson (1991) views empowerment as a process of helping people to assert control over the factors that affect their lives. This suggests that an unspecified set of conditions will be present in order for an individual to assume control. For users of mental health services, however, the factors that affect their lives include judgemental and discriminatory views and practices in the wider community that are beyond the control of individual users and individual professionals. Prejudiced social attitudes are reflected in confusion, fear and ambivalence towards users of mental health services. There is considerable doubt about society's willingness, at both an individual and a community level, to construct a culture of understanding, tolerance and acceptance. Campbell and Heginbotham (1991) describe examples of ways in which society denies users of mental health services control over their own destiny through institutionalised discrimination in housing, employment, civil liberties and health care. An individual sense of personal control over one's own life is contingent upon societal approval. Hence Gibson's approach to defining empowerment is difficult to operationalise in mental health practice.

Taylor *et al.* (1992) focus on empowerment as a political process, that is, a process involving the transfer of power. Empowerment can be seen as involving giving power *from* service providers *to* service users. Service users' own notion of empowerment does include having a stake in the control of policy making and implementation. Lindow (1993) is critical of professional power that allows a benign, professionally led agenda of what constitutes empowerment, allowing user/pressure groups filtered access to the delivery of services. She advocates empowerment through moving towards user-led services. This desired shift in power challenges mental health professionals' own power base. Lindow asks that the concept of empowerment should be operationalised through user control of the planning and delivery of services.

Lindow and Morris (1995) acknowledge that much of the public debate about empowerment takes place on the terms and in the language of those who hold the resources and those who create policy in community care. Professionals and policy makers have been the gatekeepers in containing as well as liberating individuals with mental health problems. The social control element in their role is difficult to reconcile with user empowerment. As Wright (1995) argues, the traditional professional/patient paradigm, in which knowledge is held by the professional and the patient's well-being is seen as dependent on that knowledge, is not easy to relinquish.

It is unclear whether professionals' perception of empowerment includes offering users equal opportunities in decision making. To do so would involve sharing power with those who have not traditionally had legitimate access to power. Professional power has involved not just the capacity to impose one's will, if necessary against the will of other parties, but also the power to set the terms and topics of debate and argument. Mullender and Ward (1991) are sceptical about what they call the 'Newspeak' of empowerment used by professionals. Using the language, practitioners can rewrite accounts of their practice without fundamentally changing the way in which it is experienced by service users. The term 'empowerment' can appear to create an aura of moral superiority that offers protection against criticism and attack (Mullender and Ward 1991).

Empowerment and user empowerment are many things to many people. Empowerment can be what you want it to be, depending on different agendas. Wallcraft (1994: 90) reminds us of the danger of having 'a mental blueprint of what empowerment looks like: it looks different for every individual'. The challenge for mental health workers is to acknowledge the complexities and incongruities but to work with what Mullender and Ward (1991) describe as an anti-oppressive view of care. Such a view acknowledges that users have the ability to define their own problems and to set their own agenda for change.

User empowerment in practice

Analyses of the *processes* of empowerment are ambiguous and varied. In nursing literature, empowerment is associated with coping skills, mutual support, support systems, community organisations, neighbourhood participation, personal efficiency, competence, self-sufficiency and self-esteem (Gibson 1991). Thus empowering strategies can focus either on individual competencies – empowerment as self-sufficiency – or on interpersonal links and shared needs – empowerment as mutual support or neighbourhood participation. However, there are two different foci, and the links between the two have yet to be adequately explored both in the literature and in professional practice. Such varied interpretations give little clear guide for action.

In policy and managerial analyses, examining empowerment in the context of user participation in service provision, Philpot (1994) offers a continuum of user involvement, identifying levels of user involvement. The minimum level is **information**: users are given information about services and developments. The next level is **consultation**: users' views are elicited and taken into consideration when decisions are made. More active involvement is encouraged through **partnership**: managers, professionals and users work together to plan and reach decisions about the service. The maximum level of involvement is **user control**: budgets are delegated to users to run their own services or carry out pieces of work on behalf of commissioning agencies. This framework offers mental health care workers one way in which to work progressively towards user empowerment while at the same time creating opportunities to explore substantial issues that may emerge as each of the levels of participation is implemented.

Tensions for mental health nurses: user empowerment and medical models of professional care

One of the issues that emerges in user empowerment in mental health services is the conflict of interests faced by mental health nurses and how this affects their ability to operate within medical services and yet respond effectively to users' agendas.

The neophyte nurse may have idealised views about the nature of nursing and an assumption that there is a culture of partnership between user and nurse that allows care to be negotiated by exploring and meeting individual needs. The 1982 syllabus of training for registered Mental Nurses (National Boards for England and Wales 1986) actively encouraged educationalists to deliver programmes that reflected client-centred principles, a move that suggested the importance of the individual rather than the medical condition and symptomatology. Barker (1997) reinforces this view, arguing that nurses do not have the diagnosis and treatment of mental illness as their primary concern but are more focused on identifying the mental health needs of individuals. Not only do contemporary mental health nurses argue that practitioners are no longer subservient to the medical model, but evidence from clinical practice also appears to support such claims. Sheehan (1996) identifies nursing development units as participating in promoting patient-centred methods of care and high levels of patient and relative participation in care.

This focus on meeting needs suggests user participation at a level between **consultation** and **partnership**. However, traditional models of professional practice in psychiatry are based on the development of professional–client relationships that foster trust in the medical practitioner and compliance with a treatment plan. Adopting a medical model with an emphasis on searching for problems (which clients will provide) offers clients a subservient and dependent role (the sick role, in Parsons' [1951] terms). In the sick role, patients are expected to seek medical help and accept prescribed treatment in return for exemption from normal responsibilities and for professional care and support. As a result, clients become dependent, lose control over what happens to them and come to see professionals as having the power to solve their problems. In this model, the psychiatrist, as healer, identifies the client's illness and institutes a treatment plan (Thomas *et al.* 1997). Mental health nurses carry out the treatment, usually in the form of administering medication. In such cases, the user may have no choice but to take the medication, despite concerns about dosage and long-term health effects. Rogers *et al.* (1993) indicate that users' experiences of mental health services and the care they received by medical and nursing staff was most unsatisfactory. In particular, users reported receiving insufficient information and a lack of any sense of partnership with the mental health workers looking after them.

Suggestions that the medical model acts as the main impediment to mental health nurses' ability to deliver client-centred care should, however, be challenged by raising issues about nurses' own use of power and the consequential impact on the level of user participation. As Philpot (1993) argues, practitioners bring their value judgements to their practice, for example through their perceptions of users as deserving or undeserving. Sallah (1996) describes how nurses use power when patients are secluded. Questions that need to be raised in relation to the use of seclusion include asking who benefits from the experience and what the therapeutic value for the patient might be. In practice, seclusion may be a matter of expediency in the interests of safety for the individual or others, or a consequence of professional arrogance and control.

Public concern about community safety exacerbates mental health nurses' difficulties in adopting methods of care and contributes towards a conflict for practitioners between moving towards models of care that incorporate user choice and participation, and adopting a more interventionist style of surveillance, or policing, by professionals, which moves in a direction very different from that of partnership. The evidence so far suggests that participation between users and professionals is variable in hospital settings. In practice, working in environments that are under-resourced and under-staffed, mental health nurses often tend to focus on patients' problems rather than clients' needs. There are few clients on a mental health ward who are not on neuroleptic drugs. Personal reports from clinical nurses in current care environments suggest an increasing use of medication. Although problems are best defined in the presence of the person experiencing them, problems are, in practice, often defined by professionals in an office away from the person concerned. Professionals make inferences and reach decisions *for* the person. It can be argued that, whenever professionals adopt a problem-focused approach, an important aspect of care is likely to be missed. Clients will not receive opportunities to explore available options or to participate in decision making. Denied opportunities to participate in their own care management, clients will fail to realise what they *can* do and will miss opportunities to celebrate successes when goals are reached. Success in care settings could foster confidence that could extend into relationships with other significant people in their lives.

In contrast to a problem-centred, reductionist approach, a needs-led approach can lead to holistic care. In examining what clients really need, clients are allowed to discuss what is really going on in their life and thus describe the context that could give meanings to their signs and symptoms. In negotiating their needs, the locus of decision making is shared and overt conflict is avoided. The NHS and Community Care Act 1990 aimed to facilitate such an approach.

Empowerment of users in community care settings

Simmons and Brooker (1986) argue that, for community care to be successful, it must involve not only care *in* the community, but also care *by* the community. Baron and Haldane (1992) have traced the 'positive power' of the term 'community care'. 'Community' is linked with positive images of a good life, of what is desirable and thought to promote intimacy and stability. Limpinnian (1991) challenges the link between community care and feelings of empowerment through a study of residents in a community residential home for those with enduring mental illness. He found that, although the community provided ample opportunities for integration, fewer restrictions and wider choice, service users did not find it easy to use community services. Through lack of money, the behaviour of some neighbours and ridicule by shopkeepers, the residents withdrew to where they felt comfortable and safe – the community home. The residents in the study complained of having very little purchasing power, which constrained their freedom to choose:

> You have more choices here, but you usually make the wrong choice. There are too many temptations and not adequate money (p. 63)

The poverty of residents rendered them vulnerable to economic exploitation. The manager of the residential home in the study noted that:

> the local cigarette shop is selling cigarettes in ones. The local shopkeeper has found out he can make a profit on it. (p. 63)

Not only are there economic barriers to empowerment, but there are also attitudinal barriers to integration. The manager of the home commented:

> I think they are patronised. I've had nurses hearing things that the local residents have said anti-us. They are accepted on face value but when their back is turned, they are being talked about... (p. 63)

These examples suggest that the community has preconceived ideas concerning residents' capacity to behave according to the norms of that community. Limpinnian observed that a 'resident went into the butcher's shop and the butcher said, here is another one who can't get his money out' (Limpinnian 1991: 63). These unpleasant encounters had a detrimental effect on the residents' dignity, and going out became an ordeal.

The expectation that the move towards care in the community in small residential homes would result in user empowerment derives in part from Goffman's analysis of the controlling power of total institutions (Goffman 1961). Mental hospitals were seen as typifying total institutions' ability to deny individuals control over their daily routine, a control that could be regained within smaller residential settings in the community. However, Limpinnian argues that the community home residents he studied appeared to be just as powerless in directing their own future as they were in hospitals. They appeared to be dependent on staff for many aspects of their life, including affiliation needs. Some of the residents became isolated by being unable to make new friends. In addition, some families did not want to accept the responsibility of reintegrating their family member who had been a psychiatric inpatient. One resident in the study reported, 'my husband will not have me home, he thinks I am not well enough to go home, but I think I am'. Another resident commented, 'my parents don't come and see me here'. Far from experiencing reintegration and fulfilment in the community, some residents may feel that they lose hope.

Although the care system is seeking the rehabilitation of clients, eventually into a family home, relatives may resist this. In such situations, the feelings of being unwanted could lead to a sense of helplessness and disempowerment. However, caring for a relative may not be an empowering experience for the family. Within the discourses on community care, there is an assumption that the burden of care will fall on the shoulders of the family. Families may be denied choice. As Oliver (1990) points out, whereas some families have played an active part in seeking to have their relatives discharged from long-stay hospitals, other families are now actively campaigning for institutions to remain open.

Lindow (1993) sees members of professional care teams as being engaged in obvious social control even in residential homes. Limpinnian found that many residents viewed their life as a move from one institution to another. Since the opening of the community home under study, none of the residents had been discharged home at the time of the research. There is some evidence to suggest that public education campaigns may lead to more supportive attitudes and facilitate social integration (Reid and Garety 1996, Shepherd *et al.* 1996). However, there is a need for further research into effective methods of delivering care if the community care policy is to achieve its desired outcomes.

There is limited evidence of user empowerment at the levels of **partnership** and **user control**. Interaction with mental health professionals is rarely able to counterbalance the effects of an antagonistic and discriminatory community. The involvement of users in the education of professionals is seen as one possible way to promote change in professional attitudes and beliefs towards user participation, as well as creating opportunities to explore and change the power balance between users and professionals.

The politics of education: who is the expert?

Educational programmes for mental health care professionals have recently come under scrutiny by users and/or those representing their interests. Pressure to establish user involvement in the education of mental health nurses and other health professionals have come from individuals within the user movement (Lindow 1993, Lindow and Morris 1995), government policy documents (DoH 1994, 1995, Sainsbury Centre for Mental Health 1997) as well as the professional body representing nurse education programmes in higher education (ENB 1995). *Working in Partnership* (DoH 1994) states that 'Mental Health nursing should re-examine every aspect of its policy and practice in the light of the needs of people who use services' (p. 3). More specifically, it recommends that people who use the services and their carers should participate in teaching and curriculum development. Users' involvement in the 'nurturing culture' of the trainee professional can be seen as a natural progression from policy changes, but it can also be seen as a direct challenge to the educationalist as expert. Education can be seen as a key area of influence over the future development of professionals' response to service users. Farmer (1993) argues that the mechanisms that reinforce the values of the dominant group are first and foremost educational. He argues that educational curricula play a key role in reducing conflict and supporting dominant ideas and values. Lindow

(1993) has put forward a radical agenda for changing professionals' way of perceiving users through accessing the training and educational programmes of professional groups. She criticises what she perceives as inappropriate training, particularly time spent on skills that she sees as irrelevant to users' concerns. Hopton (1995), however, points to the danger that user involvement schemes may become tokenist or involve co-opting users into relatively trivial projects that do not raise or address issues of disempowerment. An additional barrier to user input in curriculum development is mental health nurses' failure to recognise or accept that their therapeutic interventions are often perceived by clients to be oppressive.

Involvement of users in education raises important challenges to notions of professional expertise. Lindow argues that 'one key area to achieving power in moving towards user-led service will be our growing confidence in our own expertise' (1993: 184–5), suggesting that users themselves could gain 'expertise'. She seeks media recognition for this expertise, noting that 'one particular irritating characteristic of experts is the confidence with which they make their pronouncements about us. We can make equally confident and much more accurate observations. More of us can become media experts.' In similar vein, she comments, 'we want our voice to have equal weight with those of the 'experts'. We know rather more about the subject of community living in a discriminated group than they do' (pp. 184–5).

An example of this 'expert' voice in educational programmes is discussed by Carlile, who makes use of Aylott's argument that teaching sessions can be refocused to include how it feels to be on the receiving end of a nursing intervention (Carlile 1996). She describes how concepts such as empowerment and self-advocacy can be demonstrated by user involvement in the curriculum. The notion of user as educational expert, however, remains problematic. Expertise assumes attributes of skill and knowledge, attributes normally associated with professionals and often seen as being grounded in experience. Users, in claiming expert status *through* their experience as clients, are simultaneously denying and promoting claims to expertise. Both professional and client are assuming expertise in their own right. One of the parties has to retract or modify his or her own claims to expertise in order to ensure that the professional–client fiduciary relationship described by Freidson (1994) can survive. Users' claim to expertise challenges traditional notions of professionalism.

Such challenges can be relatively unproblematic for reflective practitioners as described by Schön (1983). His version of professionalism demands that professionals respect users' knowledge and accept the uncertainty of their own knowledge base. Reflective practitioners work in partnership with clients.

For educationalists, it may seem impossible to include users in the curriculum without challenging their own notion of professional expertise, grounded in the rational-legal authority of experience and qualifications. It is on this authority that the legitimacy of an apprentice/'master' model of education may be based. In addition, student nurses who have been (or are being) socialised into viewing their future professional role as essentially humanitarian may feel disempowered by tensions deriving from users presenting conflicting views that emphasise the oppressive nature of professional care. User empowerment through and within educational processes remains a issue for further exploration and critical review.

Conclusion

Putting the concept of empowerment into action remains an enormous challenge for all involved in mental health services. We have identified the potential for power struggles between professionals and users, and the possible conflicts that may inhibit the development of user empowerment strategies at the professional–user interface. Yet, as Brown argues, patients and workers share interests and experiences. Both see mental health administration as being antagonistic to their mutual interests, and both are victims of fiscal cutbacks. With respect for each other's needs, patients and ex-patients may find common goals with the mental health workforce (Brown 1993).

Mullender and Ward (1991) offer what they call a statement of practice principles, which may help in promoting a climate of empowerment as well as action by professionals. These principles include:

- working with an anti-oppressive view of care
- a belief that users have the ability to define their own problems

- users setting their own goals and taking their own action for change
- a commitment to basing action for change on a broader social analysis than is commonly the case in most professional interventions
- a style of working in partnership with people that facilitates and empowers them.

Mullender and Ward challenge both users and workers to recognise the need to share power and to use power non-oppressively. This acknowledges that there may be a transfer of power from the professional to the user.

The interface between users and educationalists has created opportunities for the seeds of empowerment to be nurtured through educational programmes for neophyte professionals. Lindow and Morris (1995) identify recommendations for training providers, including that:

- equal opportunities policies and courses should include psychiatric system survivors
- anti-oppressive training should include mental health issues
- educators should think through issues such as professionalism, boundaries and personal disclosure when introducing concepts such as user empowerment and, if necessary, question attitudes to these issues
- training in mental health should be introduced for all students, ensuring that there is more than a token input from users.

The current reality is a far cry from the above aspirations, and considerable action will be required by educationalists to move the process forward in a meaningful way.

As Morris (1993) argues, user involvement in decisions about services is an idea whose time has not only come, but is also long overdue. Barker *et al.* (1993) identifies Newcastle Mental Health Consumer Group's close working relationship with Newcastle District Health Authority as an example of good practice. The Consumer Group contributes to the purchasing of mental health services in four main ways: needs assessment, quality measures, future planning and monitoring contract performance. Lindow points out, however, that, of all the stake holders in developing appropriate community care, service users have the least money and the greatest expertise. She advocates that service users should become both purchasers and providers with the ability to buy the professional skills they find useful. They would thus provide services as part of the 'mixed economy of care' (Lindow 1993).

The real test of empowerment is the establishment of structures and processes that will demonstrate real change and benefits for users and professionals alike (Taylor *et al.* 1992). Current policies appear to have placed the interests of users firmly on the agenda, but the time scale involved suggests evolutionary rather than revolutionary change.

11 Power, knowledge and skills in child-centred care

Margaret Miers

The expectation that a sick child should have a qualified children's nurse responsible for his or her care has become a standard for care supported by *A Patient's Charter: Services for Children and Young People* (NHSE 1996). This chapter explores the nature and importance of children's nurses' knowledge and skills, and the potential gains that increasing knowledge and skill may bring to nurses and to the children and families in their care. In choosing to explore knowledge and skills, we are making some assumptions. We are assuming that nurses' knowledge and skills play a role in effective health care delivery and that, insofar as health and care are empowering for individuals, the delivery of effective health care can be seen as a process of empowerment. We also assume that the effectiveness of the *nurse* derives from the influence that he or she has on the child and family in a holistic sense *and* on the care environment.

To assume that an individual nurse has influence through knowledge and skills is to privilege certain approaches to understanding power and understanding the relationship of the individual to social structures. Power and influence are seen as part of social relationships. Individuals are 'agents' who work within 'structures' and may, through their social practices, 'make a difference' to the world in some way. These are the assumptions of Giddens' structuration theory, which links interpretative and interactionist emphases on the importance of action and meaning to 'macro' sociological approaches that emphasise the importance of social structure. Structuration theory sees structure and agency as mutually dependent; 'structural properties of social systems are both the medium and the outcome of the practices that constitute those systems' (Cassell 1993: 122). Thus professional–client relationships that can be seen as 'properties of social systems' are both the medium and the outcome of health care. The relationships are shaped by the 'structure' (organisation) of health care, but the relationships also constitute health care and in turn shape the way in which practices are organised and understood. Giddens placed power at the centre of his analysis of structuration. It is 'rules' and 'resources' that structure social practices. It is resources that can become enabling. Giddens defines power as the use of resources to secure outcomes. 'Power in this broad sense is equivalent to the *transformative capacity* of human action: the capability of human beings to intervene in a series of events so as to alter their course' (Cassell 1994: 227). In emphasising the phrase 'transformative capacity', we follow Giddens in two further respects. We acknowledge that power is not just about domination. Domination can be seen as a subcategory of relations involving power as transformative capacity. Second, we consider that zero sum theories of power are inadequate. A power gain for clients does not mean that professionals' power declines. In this chapter, we explore how children's nurses' knowledge and skills may become resources that empower *both* nurses and those in their care.

In emphasising skills and knowledge as empowering resources, we are also assuming that knowledge and skills will be resources that contribute to the nurse's legitimacy, to his or her authority. Weber's ideal types of authority (legitimate power) – traditional, rational-legal and charismatic – help to clarify differences in sources of authority. All three types of authority, however, may be reinforced, revealed and developed through a nurse's use of knowledge and skills in a relationship with a child and family. Traditional authority rests on 'traditionalism', which Weber saw as referring to the 'psychic attitude-set for the habitual workaday and to the belief in the everyday routine as an inviolable norm of conduct' (Gerth and Mills 1948: 296). Traditionalism, through, for example, patriarchal assumptions about caring females and nurses as doctors' handmaidens, can limit a nurse's role (particularly the role of a children's nurse). Nurses (or women) are not seen as responsible decision makers. Nevertheless, nurses' authority as health professionals is enhanced by traditional assumptions about nurses' (and women's) natural place tending the sick. Traditional authority can combine with the rational-legal authority brought by qualifications and state registration, bringing nurses a central role within the health care team and hierarchy.

Rational-legal authority is authority based on rules, credentials and position. Weber saw the increasing importance of rational-legal authority as a consequence of industrialisation. Industrial societies needed to develop administrative systems that were effective, efficient and rule governed in order to ensure impartiality. As rational-legal authority increased, the influence of alternative sources of authority (such as a traditional patrimonialism resulting in nepotism) diminished. The emphasis on nurses' education and qualifications brings rational-legal authority to nurses', including children's nurses', claims to expertise and professional status. The Children's Charter's (NHSE 1996) recognition of the necessary role of qualified children's nurses in health care for children and young people supports the legitimacy of specialised qualifications and thus enhances rational-legal authority.

The third source of authority that Weber identified is charismatic authority, authority that resides in 'an extraordinary quality of a person' (Gerth and Mills 1948: 295). Insofar as the knowledge and skills of a nurse, or any health care professional, involve knowledge and skills relating to communication, it is difficult to see how the potential for charismatic authority can be eliminated from health care. Charismatic authority is a resource. Children, as a social group, may be seen as possessing this resource, and children's celebration of make believe through play may mean that they are susceptible to individual charisma. The effective social practice of nursing can be seen as using, illuminating and exploring all three types of authority.

Charismatic authority is revealed in relationships, in communicative action. Rational-legal and traditional authority, while part of the relationships between individuals, are also embedded in the structure, in the organisation, of health care. Yet, as already identified, nurse–client relationships create and change structures. Rational-legal authority in health care, for example, does not have to rest with the professionals. Patients can be seen as being more knowledgeable about their own health and illness than the professionals involved in their care. Children's nurses can be seen to be in the forefront of developing family-centred care through bringing legitimacy to the role of children and their families in decision making.

An additional assumption is that focusing on *decision making* can be a fruitful way of exploring power issues. Lukes' identification of three faces of power illuminates the complexity of the power processes involved in decision making (Lukes 1974). The control of agendas (Lukes' second face) and the intricate processes that shape desires (Lukes' third face) limit or enhance the capacity of participants in any social setting to 'make a difference' through decision making. Power, in all Lukes' faces, is present in the controlling and liberating context of organisational roles and in hierarchies. Lukes' three faces of power are also at work in professional–client relationships, and the transformative power of action can work through decision making, controlling agendas and shaping desires. The consequences can be controlling or liberating. Giddens' structuration theory, Weber's types of authority and Lukes' three faces of power are varied theories and concepts that can help to explore the potential for nurses to use their skills and knowledge as empowering resources in child health care.

Child-centred care: examples for discussion

Administration of medicines

In recent years, family members have been encouraged to continue the normal daily care of their child while in hospital, and parental caring activities have been extended to include many nursing activities, such as nasogastric tube feeding. During hospitalisation, however, the responsibility for the administration of medicines has usually remained in the hands of the nurse. The hospital ward is a care setting in which, historically, power has lain predominantly in the hands of medical consultants, administrative managers and senior nurses as unit or ward managers. Control over the drugs trolley, however, has remained within the qualified nurses' domain. Legitimate control over the keys to the medicine cupboard and drug trolley ensures that drug administration remains central to nurses' work. Nurses' willingness to use drug administration to disempower through exercising control has been well documented in the literature on nursing rituals and nurses' responses to the relief of pain (Walsh and Ford 1989). On children's wards (as in other settings), if ward routine includes drug rounds, the patient may have to be awakened to receive medication (Woodhouse 1990). Nurse-led, individualised, patient-centred systems of organising care, such as primary nursing, still leave the control of medicine administration in the hands of nurses, who may have to negotiate with each other over access to the ward keys. It can be argued that only if the care system allows self-administration or, for children, gives control to a family member can sufficient flexibility be introduced to ensure that medication is available at times that are both medically appropriate and acceptable to the patient.

Woodhouse (1990) describes a change in procedures for the administration of medicines that deliberately flattens the traditional inverted hierarchical pyramid of power in ward settings, which placed the child and family at the base, their care needs supporting the professional hierarchy. The change in procedures involved an alteration in the normal pattern of administering medication within the hospital. Aware that, whatever the pattern of administration in hospital, parents would on discharge assume responsibility for their children's medication, the ward team on a paediatric oncology unit proposed that parents should be able to take responsibility for medicines while on the ward. This involved discussions with nurse colleagues, senior nursing staff, managers, medical staff, the ward pharmacist and pharmacy department, and engineers (concerning lockable storage boxes). Decisions had to be made concerning the provision, financing and location of lockable, fixed bedside medicine cabinets, the provision of individual containers of medicines and the design of a parent record chart and system of record keeping. Although many of these decisions were taken without recourse to those most affected by the decision – the children and their families – the nurses' initiative developed a system that allows parental carers to make decisions concerning medication. Parents may choose who should give medication to their child. They may choose to give control to the nurse, who may then keep the key of the medicine cabinet, but the possibility for parental involvement and for parental control has been placed on the agenda. Woodhouse (1990) concludes that 'the favourable response from parents and the control and confidence it gives them ensures that we will continue with this method of drug administration'.

Offering the family the choice of giving their child the prescribed medicines expands the range of choices that are on the agenda even though the decision making involved in prescribing remains in medical control. Thus the philosophy of partnership in care becomes part of the relationships of care and hence part of, in Giddens' terms, the 'structure'. Structuration theory assumes that the structure is created through interaction and through negotiation, in this case through decision making. There may be a transfer of power in this activity, yet what is demonstrated in the development and working of the partnership is a likemindedness of purpose, a mutuality that derives from a shared aim – to make the child's experience as free from stress as possible. Power is not so much transferred, perhaps, as shared, with the effect that both nurses' and parents' capacity to make a difference has been enhanced.

It is indeed power in the sense of 'transformative capacity' that is being exercised by the nurses, both in negotiation with individual families and in negotiation with colleagues in order to change the system. The parental administration of medicines has gained legitimacy. Beyond the hospital boundaries, however, the administration of medicines is the normal responsibility of parents. Viewed in this way, the strength and supremacy of medicalisation as a discourse is revealed. In many instances, medical control has in fact taken away control from parents. Woodhouse quotes a mother's reaction to her child's illness: 'the doctors take over and you feel totally inadequate. Lost, hopeless, stupid' (Davies, cited in Woodhouse 1990: 9). How could parental control over medication have lost its legitimacy when in a hospital setting? Asking this question exposes some of the patriarchal and traditional elements of professional claims to legitimacy, although professionals' own claims to rational-legal authority can also be reconfirmed. Expert knowledge about the action of drugs, for example, can be at the source of a claim for control in the interests of clients. Nurses' own knowledge about the importance of ensuring that medicines had been given meant that accountability remained a main issue of concern when introducing change. Accountability was shared by the prescribing doctor, pharmacist and nurse in charge of the ward (Woodhouse 1990).

If paediatric nurses are to relinquish their 'gatekeeper' role in relation to prescribed medicines, and are to do so safely, their skills in communication and interaction take centre stage. Nurses need to be able to explain to family members the nature of the medication, its rationale, its action, the mode of administration and potential side-effects. They need to be able to support and, if necessary, supervise parents who are administering medication prior to the acceptance of responsibility for their child's drugs. Children's nurses become educators and facilitators, promoting their own and others' capacity to become partners in care.

Figures 11.1–11.3 illustrate ways in which nurses' action to change the system of administration of medicines, both at organisational level and through negotiation with family members, can bring gains for nurses and for children and families. As Figure 11.1 shows, it is the nurse's communication skills that had transformative effects when attempting to change the system. The crucial role of communication skills can be seen through the range of professionals and individuals with whom the senior sister had to interact over a prolonged period of time in order to develop a workable system (Woodhouse 1990).

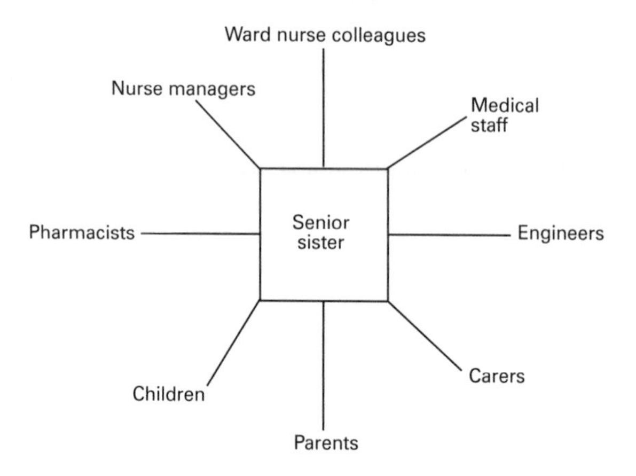

Figure 11.1 Range of professionals and individuals involved in implementing change in method of drug administration

Figure 11.2 identifies a range of potential gains for family members. These gains can extend beyond the hospital stay. When carers have received appropriate instruction and supervision prior to accepting responsibility for medicines while in hospital, increased understanding, competence and confidence can enable parents to use their enhanced knowledge when caring for a child at home. Parents increase their own knowledge and skills. In Woodhouse's study, one parent commented that 'mothers should get into a routine and not depend on the nurses too much. Nurses are not going to be at home to help them' (1990:12).

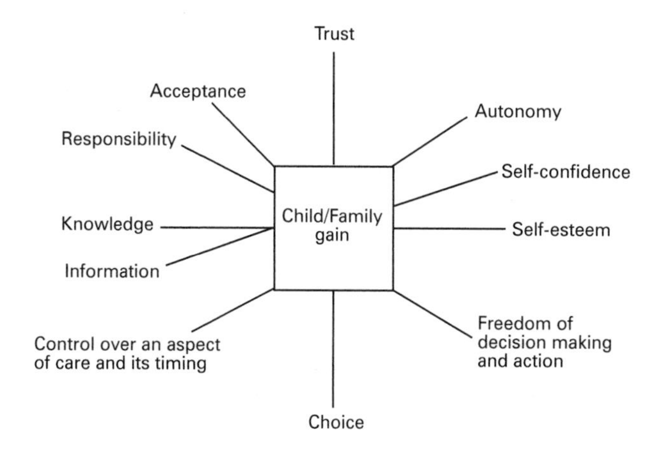

Figure 11.2 Potential gains for family members through a change in method of drug administration

Figure 11.3 illustrates a range of potential benefits for nurses. Parental administration of medicines was not an easy option. Nurses had to spend time on support and education, and identified a need for 'extra vigilance to ensure that patients receive the correct drugs' (Woodhouse 1990: 12). Nevertheless, confidence and competence gained through enhanced interdisciplinary interactions and through experience of care partnerships and shared decision making may help nurses to clarify and enhance their own role in health care teams. Nurses can gain power through increasing their influence within such teams.

There is an interesting difference between Figure 11.2, illustrating gains for child and family, and Figure 11.3, identifying gains for nurses. The gains for child and family emphasise autonomy, choice and control. The gains are individual and private. Although some gains for individual nurses may also be private and individual (confidence, knowledge), the identified gains relate to changes in

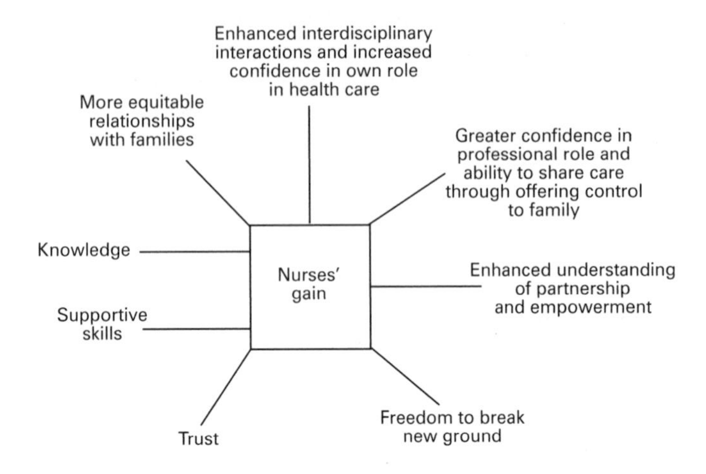

Figure 11.3 Potential gains for nurses through a change in methods of drug administration

relationships and to the nature and quality of support, trust, equity and partnership in interdisciplinary interactions and in relationships with children and their carers. 'Offering control' is a term that places enhanced human communication as the *outcome* as well as the means of nurses' own empowerment. It is possible that clients and carers gain autonomy and privacy through nurses' enhanced capacity to share responsibility for care. Collaboration may limit nurses' direct role in decision making, but it increases power to shape desires and set agendas.

Caring for abused children in accident and emergency departments

Not all families, however, provide caring environments for their children. The following account, quoted by Wheeler (1995), again illustrates the way in which an individual nurse can use knowledge and skills to 'make a difference' to a young person in her care. Sarah, a 27-year-old E-grade triage nurse in an accident and emergency department, assesses Deborah, a 13-year-old girl who presents herself with a painful swollen right wrist. Sarah suspects a Colles fracture. It is 11.30 am on a morning during school spring half-term. Sarah has recently completed the Department of Health training and study pack concerning The Children Act 1989 (DoH 1992b):

> As she is assessing her, she recognises that Deborah is very distressed and frightened. With careful questioning, Sarah finds that Deborah's stepfather is at home asleep following a night shift as a security guard. Her mother is apparently out at work... Sarah tries to get Deborah to explain how she hurt her wrist and she appears vague and mutters something about falling off her bike. At the same time Deborah appears very uncomfortable and asks for the toilet. Sarah accompanies her, and helps her with her jeans, and notices bruising to her upper thighs. On return to the cubicle, Sarah arranges priority for Deborah to be seen by the casualty registrar who is on duty that day rather than the house officer. She does this because she is suspicious that this is a non-accidental injury and wants the more experienced medical officer to examine her...
>
> ...Sarah explains to Deborah that the doctor will examine her wrist but also needs to check her body in case of other injury... Deborah is frightened and needs lots of gentle reassurance... Mark conducts the examination with Sarah in close attendance... Mark is concerned, as is Sarah, that Deborah may have been sexually abused. Deborah does not respond to any of his questions and he leaves to arrange an X-ray. As he goes, Deborah bursts into tears and holds Sarah's hand extremely tightly. Sarah asks Deborah if someone has hurt her...
>
> ...Sarah discovers that Deborah has had her wrist broken by her stepfather who came home from his night shift and tried to sexually abuse her. Deborah's mother had left for her day job.
>
> (Wheeler 1995: 58–9)

Wheeler identifies knowledge and skills that Sarah has used to enable Deborah to share information with her, thus allowing her to initiate 'the process of investigation and management in order to protect' (1995: 61). These include knowledge concerning: The Children Act 1989; the 'welfare principle' and its application; non-accidental injuries, including nurses' own difficulties in assessment; risk factors and preconditions in sexual abuse; and child protection registers and procedures for managing cases and communicating with appropriate professionals. Sarah's communication skills and ability to win trust through her presence and reassurance as well as her confidence in initiating the involvement of the registrar are noted, as is her wish to be 'an informed flexible practitioner' (p. 58) and the fact that she 'does not view nursing as a source of power and believes strongly in fostering partnership between patients and herself and the medical team' (p. 59). It is clear from the account that Sarah's communication skills are grounded in an awareness of the purpose of communication in this context and predicated on observation skills, which involve identifying cues that are both physical (bruising) and interactional (distress). Sarah also exhibits thinking skills, which involve a structured assessment and a plan of care to facilitate further assessment. (Details concerning Sarah's actions after assessment are not included in the account.) Sarah appears confident in her own skills and shows awareness of the potentially disempowering (for Deborah) nature of professional surveillance.

Sarah's application of her knowledge and skills in Deborah's assessment transforms a physical examination into a disclosure of sexual abuse. Sarah's potential gains can be identified in Figure 11.3 above. Her interactions (perhaps her status and respect) with medical colleagues may have been enhanced. She has established a sense of trust with her client and gained confidence in her abilities, which may lead her to develop new ways of working. Her discussions with other members of health and social care teams that will result from involving a multidisciplinary team in Deborah's care will further extend Sarah's experience. Sarah's communication skills, as in the earlier example, are central to the process of change and possible empowerment as identified in Figure 11.1.

However, it is difficult to place Deborah in Figure 11.2 and identify, with confidence, Deborah's gains. Deborah may have gained a sense of trust in professionals through her relationship with Sarah, and it is possible that Deborah's disclosure to Sarah, may have broken the 'power' of silence and secrecy, enhancing the confidence to say 'no'. But whether the disclosure has enhanced Deborah's self-esteem and sense of autonomy is unknown. Deborah's choice, her freedom of decision making and action, and her control over her own life remain problematic. Consequences for Deborah's relationship with her mother and for all family members are beyond Sarah's, or Deborah's, control.

The consequences of Deborah's disclosure for her mother and her stepfather are unknown. A further diagram could be drawn identifying losses for Deborah's family members and perhaps for Deborah herself.

It is evident from the example that Sarah's knowledge and skills have developed through further study, perhaps in response to increased professional emphasis on continued professional education and development. Wheeler's account of Sarah's assessment illustrates the way in which Sarah draws on her knowledge of legislation and procedures, and her knowledge of family processes that influence family functioning. It is worth considering what additional contribution a broad understanding of sociology might make to an analysis of Deborah's care.

Knowledge and skills in child-centred care: sociology's contribution

Research into student nurses' use of sociology and concepts of power in particular has identified five main categories that students use to explain the relevance of sociological study (Aust *et al.* 1996). Students identify:

1. an enhanced understanding of society,
2. an understanding of clients in broader social context,
3. an understanding of the organisational context of care,
4. identification of principles underlying care,
5. increased self-awareness and personal reflection.

Sociology could certainly enhance a nurse's understanding of broad social trends, particularly family and household trends and changes in patterns of employment. These are trends that have increased personal and financial insecurity for many children and their families. Divorce statistics suggest that at least 20 per cent of children experience parental divorce by the time they reach 16. In 1993, 55,000 children under 5 in England and Wales were affected by divorce (CSO 1996: 59).

Differing sociological perspectives provide different lenses through which to view children's circumstances and vulnerability. Feminisms, for example, may identify the complex patriarchal web of women's oppression, which can be seen as background to both sexual abuse and difficulties in disclosure. Female vulnerability can be seen as deriving from a patriarchal society. Alternatively, Marxism, suggesting economic determinism, might encourage an analysis of employment conditions that lead to families leading working lives that inhibit personal relationships. Increased awareness of different explanations for social processes that shape individual experiences may deepen recognition of the importance of providing care that takes account of the social structure and of the culture, values and beliefs of the client.

Understanding a teenage girl such as Deborah in the context of her power, or lack of it, in her own social world is to understand her vulnerability and the vulnerability of young people who cannot choose where and with whom to live. For nurses working in accident and emergency departments, however, their role in caring for abused teenagers is necessarily a limited one. Effective care will depend on collaborative work in multiprofessional teams and in partnership with families. Without skilled professional teamwork, little may be gained through a young girl's disclosure of sexual abuse to a nurse.

Conclusion

Several issues can be noted from the two examples of child-centred care. First, although nurses' skills and knowledge may 'make a difference' to the assessment, diagnosis and care of patients, whether or not such skills and knowledge become empowering resources for children and their families is problematic. Comparison of the two examples suggests that the probability of empowerment may depend on the care setting and whether or not nurses have a continuing or episodic role in client care. In accident and emergency departments, the nurses' role is limited in time and responsibility. Sarah would not have a continuing role in Deborah's care and can have no direct influence on the 'rules' and 'resources' that structure the social practices constituting Deborah's life. Nurses on a children's oncology unit, in contrast, have continuing relationships with sick children and their carers, and can thus ensure that significant aspects of care and treatment, such as drug administration, are organised in such a way as to enable families to choose appropriate modes of care. In continuing care settings, nurses may effect change in the care environment more easily.

Second, analysis of the two examples suggests that, in both episodic and continuing care settings, nurses' 'transformative capacity' depends on their ability to work constructively with other professionals. Both examples can be seen as illustrating variants of the doctor–nurse game in which nurses make suggestions that other professionals use in their own work (Stein 1967). Woodhouse, however, in publishing an account of the parental drug administration system, is publicly acknowledging nurses' leading role in initiating change. Professional teamwork can be seen as a process *in* and possibly a precondition *for* client empowerment.

Finally, the gains for child and family identified in Figure 11.2 above derive from professionals relinquishing control over drug administration and ending the ritual and routine of drug rounds. Only in the hospital setting had professionals been able to develop such a ritual. In relinquishing control, professionals are not so much giving power away as giving power *back*. What passes for client empowerment may often be described more honestly as inhibiting the process of disempowerment.

There are, however, advances in child health care that could be more significantly empowering. Caring for children on ventilators in a home environment involves the use of professional knowledge and skills in partnership with lay care and support in ways that are unprecedented in the history of medical care. Children's nurses are developing knowledge and skills that may enable them to work alongside other professionals, children, their families and other agencies, seeking freedom and opportunities to break new ground in child- and family-centred care.

The editors would like to thank Janet Edmunds-Jones for her assistance with this chapter.

12 Empowerment through sexuality

Jane Godfrey

Introduction

Nursing currently purports to offer holistic care to patients. While there may be some disagreement over what specifically constitutes holistic care, it would seem reasonable to suggest that it does include aspects of sexual identity, lifestyle and sexual health. This leads us to issues of sexuality and sexual orientation. Discussion around such issues does not feature excessively in nursing literature (James *et al.* 1994), and when it is evident, the tendency is to focus on heterosexuality as the norm. The aim within this chapter is to consider how individuals engaging with health care services may be empowered through expression of sexuality and by challenging the assumption of heterosexuality, and to identify the need for such action.

Heterosexism underpinning health care provision

Sexuality is an integral part of the whole person. To a large extent, it enables us to define ourselves. Sexuality is strongly linked with self-concept and self-esteem (Webb and Askham 1987), but it is also culturally constructed within a framework of biological, social, psychological and political needs and desires (Holland *et al.* 1990). Furthermore, Foucault (1978) argues that sexuality moved into the home with the development of the conjugal family, where it was then claimed. This has led to the identification of heterosexuality as the norm, the legitimate and therefore 'natural' sexuality. Evidence of the normacy of heterosexuality can be seen, for example, in the policies and practices that uphold the (hetero) family as the accepted unit of Western society.

The definition of heterosexuality as 'natural' has created the general assumption that all people are heterosexual. This condition, present in many societies, has been described by Rich

(1986) as 'compulsory heterosexuality' whereby women in particular are expected to behave in an heterosexual way. To be other than heterosexual is considered to be deviant. This leads to heterosexism or the belief that heterosexuality is the superior and 'proper' expression of sexuality. Even stereotypes of asexuality commonly ascribed to people who are older or disabled are centred around heterosexuality, as is the racialised sexuality of people of colour (Collins 1990, hooks 1992). The assumptions of sexuality are oppositional.

Heterosexism has been identified within health care and specifically within nursing (Jones 1988, Smith 1993, Gray *et al.* 1996) and can be seen particularly around admission/registration procedures in which individuals are required to state their marital status and family role. This can be highlighted by a quote from Stevens' (1995) study of 45 lesbians:

> When my partner was in the hospital, I was there a lot. I'd ask a question and the staff would look at me strange, like, 'Who are you? What right do you have?' Every time I had to repeat that I was a family member, her partner. (p. 27)

A further example of heterosexism may be highlighted with the immediate expectation that sexually active pre-menopausal women will need contraceptive protection to avoid pregnancy. Heterosexist practices such as these can make lesbians and gay men feel alienated from the health care process (Stevens 1992) and therefore disempowered in participating in their care. Heterosexism identifies heterosexuality as natural and superior, thereby creating and supporting a hierarchy of sexuality. Heterosexism in health care condones this general hierarchy of sexuality by making gay men and lesbians invisible as users of the services. One way of empowering users through the expression of sexuality is to listen to individuals who may experience discrimination because of their sexuality, people who do not identify as heterosexual or solely heterosexual. Such a focus immediately challenges the assumption of heterosexuality and confirms that sexuality is not necessarily always oppositional. Without such a challenge, heterosexuality continues to be invested with power through traditional authority because of its 'rightness,' and power through legal authority because it is the legitimate sexuality reinforced through social policies and practices valued in society. This power base supports heterosexist actions in institutional structures and everyday actions such as health care provision and delivery. To enable us to look at the impact of professional power and heterosexism upon users of the health service, we can consider the experiences of individuals who identify themselves as gay men or lesbians.

Power to the consumer

During the 1990s, we have seen an attempt to shift some of the power within health care provision from the provider to the user. This has been heralded through The National Health Service and Community Care Act 1990, *The Patient's Charter* (DoH 1991) and *The Health of the Nation* (DoH 1992a), which take a consumerist approach to health. Within such a framework, the user is supposedly located at the centre of health care provision. For example, *The Patient's Charter* demands that the user receive respect for their privacy, dignity and religious and cultural customs and beliefs. Furthermore, this respect should extend to relatives and friends in that information should be provided to these significant others (DoH 1991). Indeed, they may be involved in discussions regarding the planning of care for the identified user.

The Health of the Nation (DoH 1992a) adopts a broader approach but still emphasises the importance of the individual and highlights a need for feedback from the user. It also identifies a need for a focus on issues of sexual health. *A Strategy for Nursing* (DoH 1993) encourages the participation of the users of services and their carers in partnership with professionals and agencies so that individuals are enabled to achieve and maintain optimal physical, psychological and social well-being when they and/or their carers cannot achieve this without assistance. The user is, then, expected to participate in the process of health maintenance, and this is confirmed by the requirements made of nurses.

The UKCC describes the duty that nurses have to:

> work in an open and co-operative manner with patients, clients, and their families, foster their independence and recognise and respect their involvement in the planning and delivery of care

and to

> recognise and respect the uniqueness and dignity of each patient and respond to their need for care, irrespective of their ethnic origin, religious beliefs, personal attributes, the nature of their health problems or any other factor
>
> (UKCC 1992b)

again reinforcing the centrality of the individual as consumer in health care provision. The assumption is that the consumer role is a useful one for the individual to adopt. However, James and Gabe (1996) argue that this may at times create uncertainty and emphasise a user's vulnerability.

Personal responsibilities for health

The centralising of the consumer can be seen to encourage increased personal responsibility for health care decisions. Within this ethos of personal responsibility, Salsberry (1993) notes three differing interpretations highlighted by Wickler (1987). The first is that an individual's behaviour will have a primary effect on his or her health. The health care system only intervenes as a secondary source in the achievement of health. The second interpretation suggests that, as lifestyle choices can affect health, making individuals responsible will encourage them to make 'wise' lifestyle choices. The third interpretation links responsibility to cause and effect – individuals are held responsible for their illness because of certain actions or practices.

Any of these interpretations insists than an individual's lifestyle will impact on his or her health. This concept is reinforced through health education campaigns in which health care workers are involved. Nurses and other health care workers therefore need an understanding of a range of lifestyles to participate in this system of health care provision, especially if they are to avoid using these interpretations in a discriminatory way of blaming the victim.

In looking more closely at Wickler's interpretations of personal responsibility for health, it is possible to argue that, within a framework of heterosexism, there is a lack of equity in how the three approaches may be used. Lesbians and gay men who experience homophobia and discrimination may do so because they are trying to live in a manner that is 'open' and 'honest' and health promoting. They are not necessarily able to challenge discrimination that may have a profound and continuing affect on their health. For example, Taylor and Robertson (1994) report that ageing gay men who 'come out' experience ridicule and ostracism. Many older people experience isolation; if this is further reinforced through discrimination and prejudice, the health of ageing lesbians and gay men will be jeopardised. Attempting to confront heterosexism may in itself be health-harming for the individual in terms of stress, fear and anxiety. To then engage in a health care service that reinforces that very same heterosexism may also be health-harming in similar ways. Wickler's first interpretation is inadequate within a structure where heterosexuality is seen as superior and natural.

In the second interpretation, whereby the individual is responsible for making 'wise' lifestyle choices, the question that needs to be asked is, what constitutes a wise choice? A wise choice in a homophobic society may be to be silent about one's sexuality. If individuals experience less direct homophobia by remaining closeted or secretive about their sexuality, this may be a positive adaptation. However, such a position may be quite detrimental to health if these same individuals are then in a situation in which they have to lie or be deceitful in some other way. Taylor and Remafedi (1993) provide an example of a 17-year-old who was suffering from vague illnesses and hence missing school. He eventually decided to talk to the school nurse, expressing his loneliness and expecting to be laughed at when he 'came out'. He was surprised to be taken seriously. He was living with heterosexism and trying to live 'wisely'. Within a framework of heterosexism, wise lifestyle choices can be problematic.

The third interpretation that Wickler identifies is the cause and effect approach. In this, individuals are considered to have responsibility for their health in that their behaviour affects their health directly. A situation that is not uncommon for lesbians and gay men is one in which it is assumed, particularly within mental health services or psychotherapy, that the cause of illness or disturbance is the individual's sexual orientation (Platzer 1990, Taylor and Robertson 1994). This is seen particularly in relation to gay men and HIV-positive status. Gay men are rarely portrayed as innocent victims and may be seen by some as deserving what they get.

Taylor and Robertson (1994) report Synoground and Kellmer-Langan's (1991) claim that 30 per cent of nurses infer that gay men will have AIDS. Thus the cause and effect approach can be seen to dismiss completely the effects of heterosexism generally on individuals. As such, it is possible to argue that the current shift in responsibility for health from society to the individual can actually be disempowering for gay men and lesbians because of the structures and processes of heterosexism and homophobia.

To assume that the shift of power from provider to user can happen in full may be naïve for, as Hugman (1991) states:

> the caring professions can be seen to exercise power not only through skilled practices which meet the needs of their clientele but also through state sponsorship... that provides the institutional basis for those practices. (p. 29)

Nurses and other health care staff have sometimes conflicting responsibilities – those to the employing organisation and those to the user. Such conflict may help to maintain the *status quo*, thereby ensuring that power does not shift. It may be more important for an individual worker to remain in employment than to risk dismissal by pursuing an issue of advocacy for the user. Employers may utilise power in such a way as to ensure that staff acting as advocates for patients are not heard or taken seriously. Arguably, this happens when nurses suggest that they are not able to provide adequate care for users because of a lack of staff. If extra funds are not available, Lukes' (1974) second face of power may come into force, and discussion of quality of care may be kept off the agenda, leading to an obvious conflict of interest between employers and employees.

Alternatively, employers may use training and managerial influence to shape the desires of health care workers. Such an example can be seen in the focus of individualised care, in which individualised care does not acknowledge differences between people. This can lead to the common claim, 'I treat everyone in the same way.' Workers may believe that they can offer truly individual care by treating everyone the same, but everyone is not the same, and some are already more or less privileged than others, yet such workers may have been particularly influenced by messages from managers and other workers that this is the policy of the institution. So, Lukes' third face of power may be identified here, where staff beliefs are shaped according to the values of the executive of the organisation. Is this a shifting of power?

Power – shifting or static?

In fact, it is possible to argue that the power has not shifted at all – it only appears to be shifting. What may be changing is the language that has 'reproduced and communicated' that power (Hugman 1991: 37) so that users are being involved in their care but the expectation is still that they will 'co-operate' with the professional carer. If this is the case, how might we access this information? One approach would be to consider reported experiences of users as a means of developing a body of knowledge that reflects the impact of professional power as felt by consumers. This may help to increase the visibility of an often unacknowledged power base within nursing, to facilitate improved communication between users and professional carers, and to enable some sense of partnership in care.

There is an increasing amount of literature becoming available on the health experiences of lesbians and gay men, although much of this originates in the United States. While it is important to recognise that not all gay people will have identical experiences, it is valuable to highlight factors that may empower this group to use health care services in a more effective way. This, in itself, can help to improve such services for all men and women as power issues that lie hidden in taken-for-granted assumptions are challenged and health care staff are encouraged to acknowledge and analyse the effects of dominant values and beliefs upon the organisation and delivery of care. So, although the literature from America may not always be totally pertinent within the British health care system, there will be general principles that we can apply in the United Kingdom. In the meantime, we need to conduct research studies (such as that currently being carried out by the RCN) in the United Kingdom to develop a body of knowledge and concomitant actions that facilitate partnership in care for gay men and lesbian users of health care services. Perhaps then, we can say that power is shifting.

How do gay men and lesbians experience health care provision?

In exploring the experiences of this group, it is essential to set the scene of 'deviance'. Lesbians and gay men are generally devalued and disempowered through the 'deviancy' of their sexuality. Openly gay men and women, and others who may appear to be gay or gay-friendly, experience hostility and discrimination in everyday life (Stevens and Hall 1988). Ironically, this homophobia can have deleterious effects on the health of individuals who may also internalise such negative attitudes and values. This may result in an individual experiencing feelings of self-hatred, self-contempt and guilt, through their sexuality (Irwin 1992, Gilbert 1993, Nelson 1997). This is usually referred to as an internalised homophobia and can have a very controlling effect on an individual. Many gay men and lesbian users identify fear and difficulties around disclosing their sexuality to health care workers (Hitchcock and Wilson 1992, Taylor and Remafedi 1993, Stevens 1994). If this is coupled with internalised homophobia, the magnitude of avoiding disclosure and maintaining a story of lies is highlighted.

Disclosure is one of the first issues of concern for the users who are lesbian or gay. How much information about their sexuality do they need to reveal, and what responses may they get from health care staff? Linked with this issue of disclosure is confidentiality. For some, 'coming out', or revealing their sexual identity to hospital staff, may create a fear of exposure to others. Alternatively, disclosure may provide an individual with a sense of control and reduce stress (Stevens and Hall 1988). Hershberger and D'Augelli (1995) report that, for young people, 'coming out' may be linked with their fear of losing friends and being rejected by their family. There is often a lack of support in exploring sexual issues (Taylor and Robertson 1994, Nelson 1997). That this group also has a higher rate of attempted suicide suggests that care should be taken to avoid accidentally 'outing' young people to their families. The importance of confidentiality is obvious around issues of sexuality and disclosure. 'Outed' lesbians and gay men may experience discrimination, for example in employment, housing and child custody, purely on the grounds of their sexual orientation (James *et al.* 1994). Some experience violence. Torensen (1995) writes of a man admitted to an accident and emergency department following an incident of 'queer-bashing', and Stevens (1995) quotes a lesbian mother who feared violence from the child's father if he discovered that she was in a same-sex relationship.

Another factor that has been reported to affect disclosure is the response of health care workers. Many lesbians and gay men have experienced, or anticipate, negative responses from health care workers (Hitchcock and Wilson 1992, Eliason 1993, Rose 1993, Stevens 1994, Taylor and Robertson 1994). For some, this acts as a deterrent to seeking health care, and individuals may experience deteriorating health while they delay engaging in health care services (Zeidenstein 1990). Others report positive responses to disclosure (Stevens 1994), but fear of discrimination means that disclosure is fraught with uncertainties.

The reported attitudes of health care staff include a wide range of behaviours. Most commonly identified responses tend to be negative and discriminatory. This is, perhaps, not surprising as we are all affected by socialisation processes, but it does highlight the need for awareness of prejudice in health care workers. Prejudicial responses can disempower individuals, particularly when they originate from people in professional and respected positions.

Roberts and Sorensen (1995) report hostile behaviour, including pity and disgust, with a general assumption of heterosexuality. This assumed heterosexuality is further reported in the study by James *et al.* (1994), who also document the fact that gay men and lesbians are sometimes seen as a sexual threat. Some health care workers appear to be fearful that an individual may make sexual advances (James *et al.* 1994) or assume that all gay men present a high risk of HIV, 'placing "high risk" stickers on everything from TPR charts to the drip chambers of giving sets for intravenous fluids' (Irwin 1992: 435). Scandlyn (1988) suggests that gay men with HIV/AIDS are seen as guilty because of the construction of AIDS, whereas heterosexual people contracting HIV are more likely to be considered innocent victims (unless they are drug users). Ironically, Koetting (1996) describes the 'survivor guilt' that some HIV-negative gay men experience – another example of internalised homophobia providing a mirror image of societal homophobia.

Other reported behaviours include an inability to say the word 'lesbian' (Hall 1994), a partner being overlooked, a curt manner, avoiding touch, poor eye contact, minimal attention, shaming (Stevens 1994), lesbian women being refused obstetric intervention, rough physical handling, poor communication and lack of a safe environment for disclosure (Stevens 1992, Fairchild *et al.* 1996).

Reported positive behaviours include good communication skills, warmth and sensitivity, compassion (Stevens 1994) and being cared for by gay and lesbian staff (James *et al.* 1994). Lesbians and gay men need to feel accepted and valued rather than pathologised by their sexuality. Lesbians participating in Stevens and Hall's (1988) study were looking to be treated in a way in which their sexual orientation was taken calmly and as a matter of fact, their partners being included without challenge. Such responses from health care workers show support and respect. Positive behaviours are reported less frequently than negative ones but can be seen to be empowering when they are used.

Other experiences that discourage disclosure and involvement in care relate to safety. Taylor and Robertson (1994), among others, report a fear of physical harm, while James *et al.* (1994) identify fear of the consequences of being identified as gay or lesbian. These fears may be exacerbated by previous negative encounters with health care workers (Hitchcock and Wilson 1992) and highlight the potency of discrimination and ignorance in those same workers. The taboo of sexuality in Western society leads to lesbians and gay men being made invisible (Hall 1994) unless they are prepared to announce themselves, and, having announced themselves, they may then become the focus of discrimination through a lack of knowledge and understanding on the part of the health workers. Stevens (1994) documented 332 episodes of lesbians interacting with health care workers – of these, only 23 per cent were positively evaluated. Clearly, disclosure can be health-harming.

Another aspect that may contribute to fear and feelings of powerlessness among this particular group concerns family relationships. Heterosexual relationships and families often have legal status and are supported by governmental policies. Same-sex co-parents do not have this formal support; neither do lesbian mothers always enjoy legal support or protection (Stevens 1995). In fact, same-sex relationships are, at times, actively devalued by the legal system. Within the United Kingdom, for example, Section 28 of the Local Government Act 1988 prohibits the promotion of homosexuality and describes same-sex family groups as 'pretend' families. To be so discredited by the legal system does little to empower; neither does it engender confidence. This is reflected in interviews conducted by James *et al.* (1994) showing that lesbian and gay parents fear that children may be taken away from them if health care workers do not maintain confidentiality following the disclosure of sexual orientation.

Same-sex couples have repeatedly reported that partners or lovers are not always given the same respect or attention that a heterosexual partner would receive. Individuals can experience increased isolation if their partner is excluded or ignored by health care workers, or if their 'legal' next of kin demands priority over their partner. Once again, the privileging of heterosexuality is highlighted.

The assumption of heterosexuality means that inappropriate health care or information may sometimes be given. For example, women who do not have penetrative sex with men may be given information on contraceptive issues (Stevens 1994). However, the converse is also true. Stereotypical ideas about gay men and lesbians might be adopted. Examples include assuming that gay men and lesbians never have sexual relationships with members of the opposite sex, that being gay or lesbian is a mental health issue for the individual (Trippet 1994), that lesbians do not need cervical smears and that to have a same-sex sexual orientation is a phase (Taylor and Remafadi 1993).

The available literature shows that lesbians and gay men do experience discrimination and homophobia within health care arenas. Discrimination reduces individuals' opportunity to assert themselves and be heard; homophobia may be internalised and engender shame and self-contempt. Such behaviours, thoughts and feelings may be detrimental to health. If the gay or lesbian client is to be central in the health care process, an environment must be created that ensures acceptability and confidentiality. Such an environment may then enable the specific health needs of this group to be acknowledged. Living with homophobia may lead to an increased incidence of alcohol abuse (Hall 1994, RCN 1994a), depression (Trippet 1994), 'queer-bashing' and other forms of violence, poor self-esteem and an increased risk of suicide, particularly in young people (Hershenberger and D'Augelli 1995, Torensen 1995). By addressing these needs for this group, care can be improved for all people in that individuals are valued for their differences rather than without them. By valuing individuals, health care workers can empower people to care about themselves and thus promote mental health.

Empowerment through issues relating to sexuality

A useful starting point is to consider gay and lesbian users as 'outsiders within'. This concept argues that people who are 'different' view everyday practices and dynamics from a different perspective (Collins 1990). Because health care practices are entrenched in heterosexist policies, gays and lesbians are able to highlight and challenge some of the assumptions that are made and promoted through the organisation and delivery of care. 'Outsiders within' can bring a new awareness and knowledge to the health care process, and the development of this knowledge can provide users with a firm base from which partnership in care can grow. First, health care workers must listen to the voices of lesbian and gay health care users.

The King's Fund has considered ways of increasing user participation (1995). One way to do this is to encourage specific user groups to discuss health care needs with health care providers. This would create an arena that is currently occluded by heterosexism. Lesbian and gay users would have some space within which to speak at a public level; this would represent an opportunity to develop trust between user and provider built on direct communication (James and Gabe 1996).

In order to provide appropriate care, health care workers have a responsibility to inform themselves of pertinent health issues around sexuality: What are the alternatives to heterosexuality? How do people build relationships when there are no traditional structures such as marriage to support and confirm relationships? What are the specific health care needs of gay men, lesbians, bisexuals and transgendered people for example? That many health care workers appear to lack such knowledge suggests that what is considered to be appropriate knowledge within health care provision (that is, what *is* known) is only relevant for a section of the population. Gay men and lesbians need to see their knowledge and themselves reflected in the health care process. Bidwell (1988) reveals the importance for mental health of enabling young people to have easy access to literature concerning gay and lesbian issues. The same is true for adults, and there is a need for health literature that reflects the experiences and knowledge of this group.

In effect, the invisible need to be made visible and to be valued. This can be achieved through nursing research that focuses on this group and through improvements in assessments of users' needs. The assessment process often assumes heterosexuality, and there is a need to use more open questions such as: Who are the important people in your life? Are you in an established relationship? Who would you like informed about your admission? Do you have any childcare responsibilities? Questions like these do not make assumptions about people's roles or relationships and help to create an environment that does not demand conformity. This process can be facilitated to some degree by the use of frameworks for assessment that are not steeped in heterosexual assumptions, and by using the nursing process, which leads to evaluation of care.

Another aspect of care that can lead to empowerment is good communication. Studies have been referred to where care was evaluated positively because health care workers demonstrated good communication skills. Those most appreciated seem to revolve around empathy and listening. Some aspects of gay and lesbian relationships may be difficult to describe because of inadequate language. Eliason (1993) suggests that this can be disempowering – how do a same-sex couple refer to one another – partner, lover, friend? Health care workers need to listen and hear such terms and reflect them back. Empathetic listening can be used to develop a relationship of trust and provide validation for same-sex relationships (Nelson 1997).

In order to develop good communication with this group of users, health care workers may find it useful to reflect on their own ideas about sexuality and to consider in what ways they perpetuate heterosexism. How often is the assumption of heterosexuality made? Does someone have to look like a 'dyke' or a 'queen' if they are lesbian or gay? Gay men and lesbians are present in all areas of health care as workers – are these individuals able to speak about themselves without fear of discrimination? An awareness of one's own behaviour, thoughts and feelings is an important element of communication and is essential if health care workers are to support lesbian and gay users by challenging heterosexism and homophobia (Gray *et al.* 1996). Platzer (1990) reports that attitudes can also be positively influenced if lesbian and gay groups are involved in teaching.

Before being able to challenge heterosexism, health care workers need an understanding of the issues pertinent to health care and an awareness of how discrimination is perpetrated. As workers gather such knowledge, they will be able to provide general support to individuals (Deevey 1990), show solidarity with users (Stevens 1994) and possibly improve the level of awareness of gay and lesbian issues within health care. By recognising and acknowledging the effects of living in an often hostile environment, health care workers can begin to create a safer space for all people of minority groups.

The main actions that can enable workers to empower lesbians and gay men as they engage in the health care process relate, then, to knowledge, communication, self-awareness and behaviours. Health care workers who inform themselves on gay and lesbian issues can create an environment that provides opportunities for safe disclosure; good communication skills can be used to enhance that safe environment and promote trust and confidentiality; self-awareness can make health care workers more attuned to their ideas and beliefs and promote honest interactions; and a knowledge of local and national support services for gay men and lesbians can show an acceptance of gay and lesbian people. These actions can lead to positive behaviours that identify and challenge heterosexism and homophobia, thereby allowing lesbians and gay men to participate in their care as partners with health care workers. Empowerment is possible through the expression of sexuality when heterosexism is challenged.

The actions identified need to be supported within educational structures. Heterosexism needs to be identified within curricula. A radical suggestion for change would be the problematising of heterosexism in health care provision at institutional and individual levels. However, such action would constitute major change and requires protracted political action. Curriculum changes that might be useful could include the incorporation of research focusing on lesbian and gay health; an expansion on definitions of the family, with the acknowledgement of the 'normal' family being founded within heterosexuality; identification of the limitations of language in relation to family form (for example, children living with their biological mother and her co-parenting partner might say that they have two mothers); the identification of language as potentially disempowering; and the explication of the processes of oppression as they affect any minority group.

The implications of these suggestions are broad ranging, but it has been shown that lesbian and gay health care users express high levels of dissatisfaction with the service, and that by taking action that challenges heterosexist practices, health care workers can empower this group in the expression of sexuality. Changes improving services to this group will lead to overall improvements in services to all people.

The chapter also raises many questions. What is the role of the individual health care worker in challenging heterosexism if the institution does not acknowledge heterosexism? How can we begin to develop policies that do not assume heterosexuality? Is it possible to empower individuals when the priorities of the institution are constrained by finance? How can gay and lesbian workers be empowered within the structures of health care provision? Is the shifting of power merely rhetorical, in the sense that staff express the desire to provide individualised care but do not actually allow user involvement because of an unspoken rule that users will *conform* in their care? There is a need to value diversity and use difference as a tool for empowering health care users and for creating partnerships in care that enable specific care to be provided.

13 Involving clients in decision making: breast care nursing

Margaret Miers

Introduction

The importance of involving patients in decisions concerning care and treatment is now acknowledged through policy, public and professional initiatives. NHS reforms have sought to offer choice in health care services through the development of an internal market. Public pressure groups such as the UK National Breast Cancer Coalition stress the importance of service users playing a full role in decisions about relevant issues (Air 1996). Professional recognition of the ethical importance of autonomy and self-determination has been reinforced by legal attention to the importance of informed consent (Sutherland *et al.* 1989). In Sidaway *v* Governors of the Royal Bethlem Hospital and others, 1984, the House of Lords rejected Mrs Sidaway's claim of negligence for failure to warn of a 1 per cent risk of damage to her spinal cord, but encouraged doctors to give serious consideration to patients' information needs and to doctors' professional duty to inform (Brahams 1985). The nursing profession, through the UKCC *Guidelines for Professional Practice* (1996), now recognises the importance of adequate information in gaining clients' consent. The *Guidelines for Professional Practice* section on client advocacy and autonomy acknowledge the importance of recognising a patient's or client's right to choose, respecting the choices made and the right to take part in decisions about care (UKCC 1996: 13–14).

This chapter explores issues surrounding client involvement in decision making through reviewing nurses' involvement in the care of women with breast cancer. It asks whether changes in approaches to decision making involve changes in power relations and explores the effects of common assumptions and practices in care settings on the decision process itself. Nurses' role in facilitating participation in decision making has now gained widespread acceptance, at least in the rhetoric of nursing literature (Manthey 1980, Wright 1986, James and Biley 1989, Biley 1992). Breast care nurses have been at the forefront of identifying the importance of nurses' role in information giving and facilitating informed choice. The Royal College of Nursing Breast Care Nursing Society's Standards of Care (RCN 1994b), for example, prioritise 'information' and 'treatment choice' as topics 1 and 2 in the list of 9 standards.

Lukes' three faces of power could provide one starting point for an analysis of nurses' role in involving patients in decision making. Participating in treatment decisions appears to offer women an opportunity to exercise the first face of power. However, as Lukes (1974) makes clear, even when we are offered an opportunity to exercise power through decision making, we may not have influence or control over the range of options on offer. Indeed, we may not be aware of the range of options. Women rarely have any control over choices on the agenda. They do not exercise the second face of power. Furthermore, women may be asked to make a choice between options at a time when the opportunity to clarify and identify their own preferences is limited. Women may not be aware of the exercise of the third face of power, which may be shaping desires through shaping perceptions of who they are, how they should look and how they are likely to feel.

Foucault's analysis of the relationship between power and knowledge and the importance of medical discourses in framing analysis and action in daily life helps to illuminate power relationships and processes in all three faces of power. Foucault's (1976) work on the development of medical knowledge shows how observation, through the clinical gaze, led to a form of seeing and saying that linked signs and symptoms to diseases and led to the dominance of clinical discourse in medical decision making. Involving patients in decision making takes place within a medical discourse about disease, treatment and survival. Involving clients in decision making emphasises the importance of patient preferences, but agendas and desires are nevertheless still framed in and by discourses about disease, about knowledge and about men and women's lives.

Power relations, information and decision making

Control over decision making can be seen as an intrinsic part of professional dominance. Professional dominance rests on professional knowledge. Professions are, in Katz's terms, 'traditional guardians of bodies of knowledge' (Katz 1969: 55). Doctors control decision making in health care because they are presumed to have relevant knowledge and information, on which the decision must be based. Traditionally, doctors, nurses and patients accepted 'the physician as the ultimate guardian of knowledge about the patient's illness' (Katz 1969: 55). Current acceptance of the importance of *giving* information still implicitly accepts that the information belongs to the professionals. It is theirs to give away. Nurses, in facilitating information giving, are mainly supporting medical power. Doctors make decisions on the basis of information gained from various sources, including medical research, clinical examinations, laboratory tests, a patient's medical history and reported symptoms. The decisions that doctors make involve choosing between options – courses of action – that may or may not lead to particular outcomes. In breast cancer, the outcomes to be considered are those which women may have difficulty thinking about – loss of a breast, loss of life.

These outcomes may be more or less probable and, in addition, more or less desirable. Using the terms of decision analysis, the outcomes have probabilities and utilities (Miers 1990). In order to make an informed choice between options, it is important to have information concerning the probability (likelihood) and utility (desirability) of the different possible outcomes. Choosing between options therefore involves a range of sources of information. Who decides depends on who has control over sources of information and methods of presenting and collecting that information.

Doctors have information about probabilities (likelihoods) of treatment outcomes. Such information comes from national and international research studies. Treatment options are offered to women when the probabilities of successful disease control through one method are considered to be equal to those using another method. Women are therefore offered choice when the 'best' course of action is not clear. Explaining treatment options involves acknowledging openly the probability not only of success, but also of failure. Explaining treatment options involves acknowledging the limits and uncertainty of medical knowledge. Doctors do not know, with certainty, the disease trajectory for individual women. Nor do they know an individual woman's preferences concerning types of treatment or a woman's feelings about the accompanying side-effects. The utility (desirability) of possible outcomes cannot be identified without consulting the women themselves. Involving women in decisions about breast cancer treatment thus involves two-way professional–client information *exchange*. Women need information from professionals, but professionals need information about the women themselves.

Knowledge about women, as opposed to their disease, has not, traditionally, been a medical priority. Nurses have been well placed to gain information about patients as individuals. In the doctor–nurse game identified by Stein (1967), it is this knowledge about individuals which informs the recommendations concerning treatment that nurses make without, as Stein argued, 'appearing to'. Nurses are expected to play a key role in presenting information to the patient and in facilitating information exchange between doctors and patients. The exchange of information between nurses and clients can be central to decision making. If treatment options do have similar probabilities of a 'successful' outcome (usually measured by survival rates over periods of time), the choice is often made on the basis of women's preferences. Breast care nurses see themselves as enabling women to identify and express their preferences. Women are asked, for example, to think about, among other things, surgery to remove a breast or part of their breast tissue, about impaired mobility in an arm after axillary node clearance, about tolerating nausea and about regular visits to a hospital for radiotherapy and/or chemotherapy. Involving clients in decision making has the potential to alter relationships within the health care team and significantly change the balance of power. Nurses can play a key role in negotiating such changes through enabling patients to exercise the first face of power and make their own decisions. Nevertheless, although women may have a choice of treatment, they have little control over the treatment choices on the agenda. National variations in treatments and treatment choices for breast cancer have been a topic of concern (Calman and Hine 1995).

Organisational constraints on patient involvement in decision making

Clinical surveillance

Katz (1969) noted that, whereas professionals are the guardians of bodies of knowledge, knowledge is harnessed and created in social organisations. The hospital developed in an age of high regard for science, and although it harnessed 'both scientific and non scientific resources for the care and treatment of patients', the nurturant care of the nurse took a low place in the hospital hierarchy (Katz 1969: 56). Hospitals, as Foucault's (1976) work has helped to clarify, remain organised in ways that privilege the information sources on which medical knowledge is based.

Sociological accounts of hospital and clinic settings have illuminated the powerlessness of the patient, a powerlessness reinforced through the 'ceremonial order of the clinic' (Strong 1978), patients often being literally and figuratively 'stripped of their identity' (Goffman 1961). While doctors collect the information necessary for them to demonstrate their professional expertise through exercising professional judgement, women are subjected to a disempowering gaze, as one woman's account describes:

> I felt terrible; I was scared stiff and shaky and really embarrassed lying there on the examination couch with just this flimsy gown that didn't cover me right up. He came in with a couple of young doctors, and oh I was so ashamed, the way he examined me – I've got such big breasts you see. He just didn't seem to act as though I was there and kept talking to the others about the difficulty in knowing what to do with big breasts. I asked him what was wrong with me. He said 'You must realise it's cancer; we'll have you in next week sometime' and walked out.
>
> (Fallowfield 1991: 43)

Foucault's (1976) work on the power of medical discourse through the development of the clinical gaze can help to illuminate the way in which surveillance of the body is part of the institutionalisation of medical control. It is also intrinsic to the collection of information, to diagnosis and to the development of medical knowledge. Doctors have power over women through their knowledge about the disease, gained through the clinical gaze. It is an intrusive and disempowering gaze. Women's breasts are observed, manipulated and classified as diseased. Fox (1993) discusses the power of the medical profession in terms of the power to inscribe the body with meaning:

> The description of the body which medicine deciphers in its examinations, is not straightforward, it cannot be 'read' correctly by just anyone: the reader must be an *expert*. And consequently, this expertise is achieved at the expense of those who must be subjected to the power of the gaze.
>
> (Fox 1993: 29)

The diagnosis of breast cancer is an exemplar of the expertise that the profession of medicine develops through many 'ways of looking' – through palpation, through fine needle aspiration, through X-ray, all explorations of women's breasts that give to others a 'knowledgeability' (Nettleton 1992, Fox 1993) denied to women themselves. Paradoxically, clinical knowledge gained for the benefit of women has been gained through a process of disempowerment. Sharing that knowledge with women may reduce the imbalance of power.

Nurses may be able to help to reduce this imbalance. Women may be asked to make decisions, but they may have little control over the options available or over the setting or timing of their decision. Both setting and timing can be disempowering. Breast care nurses may be able to help to prevent depersonalisation and loss of dignity, which can seem an intrinsic part of clinical surveillance but without which early and accurate diagnosis would be difficult if not impossible. The importance of ensuring that women learn about the diagnosis when fully clothed, accompanied by a friend or partner, is not just an issue of dignity and respect. It is a recognition of the importance of minimising the inscriptive power of the clinical gaze. Good practice in communicating the diagnosis involves the presence of the breast care nurse, the provision of a separate room for further discussions and the presence of a friend or partner if so desired by the patient. Nevertheless, communicating test results remains the responsibility of the doctor, who fits it into his or her work routine in a way that is rarely questioned. One breast care nurse, however, commented:

> Personally I think it would be nice if he was the one that got up and went out of the room and left us to talk it through rather than us taking the patient out and looking for another room.
>
> (SSRU 1994: 35)

Timing of diagnosis

As with the setting in which women are asked to make a decision, the timing of the decision is often beyond women's control. Women with breast disease may find that they are offered an opportunity to make their own decision concerning treatment at a time when the stress of the diagnosis makes it difficult to think clearly. Many women who learn that they have breast cancer, particularly if detected through mammographic breast screening, feel healthy and are shocked by the diagnosis. A 45-year-old business woman, diagnosed after a routine examination at a Well-Woman clinic, recalled:

> I suppose that was the most difficult thing to accept. I felt so well and yet the cancer had been there for some time. I felt as though my body had let me down and I couldn't trust it any more.
>
> (Fallowfield 1991: 73)

Breast care nurses thus have opportunities to facilitate women's use of the first face of power at a time when women feel a loss of control over the agenda and when they face, perhaps for the first time, a serious threat to their health, their life, their body and their family and relationships. Lesley Thompson, former chair of RCN Breast Care Nursing Society, describes a consultation when a woman receives a cancer diagnosis as a crisis situation and notes:

> In a crisis situation... the helper has two and a half minutes to make the right impression. If she fails in this she becomes part of the problem rather than a way towards finding a solution.
>
> (Thompson 1994)

Taking control

In telling her own story, Joyce Wadler, an American journalist, gives an account of her own quest to control her experiences (Wadler 1992). She chooses doctors, clinics, hospitals, treatment and friends to accompany her through consultations. The American system of health care may provide greater opportunities for control through differing approaches to what Biley has termed the 'organisational constraints' that can inhibit (and encourage) participation in decision making (Biley 1992). Care systems in which women do choose their own specialists and have a choice of appointment dates and times may in themselves facilitate feelings of control. Nevertheless, nurses can help women to control aspects of their care within the NHS. Some breast care nurses describe efforts to encourage women to deal with their own difficulties with NHS appointment and organisational procedures as efforts to facilitate autonomy. The SSRU research reports one breast care nurse as saying:

> I help them to make appointments and with things they find stressful about the hospital, and I try to empower them to deal with the system in any way that they feel comfortable with.
>
> (SSRU 1994: 56)

'Dealing with the system' is a problem not just for patients, but also for staff. The communication settings remain controlled by the dominant medical profession and are constrained by the accepted mode of organisation of health care, which in Britain may still remain a system in which client (and nurse) remains passive. The SSRU study showed that both women and nurses regretted the nurses' lack of time available to spend with women. The setting in which communication and decision making takes place often remains a setting in which both nurse and client are disempowered. The control that the medical profession retains over the communication settings is reflected in women's assumptions about roles in the health care team. Women have had difficulty understanding the role of specialist nurses, often confusing them with members of the medical team. The SSRU report notes that 'one woman described having helpful information from "I think she was an anaesthetist who was just filling in time"' (SSRU 1994: 50). Nor are all breast cancer nurses perceived as helpful – 'she wanted me to hold her hand when they put the needle in, but I would rather have held my own hand and squeezed it hard' (SSRU 1994: 50). Despite research that shows the benefits of specialist support (McArdle *et al.* 1996), only about half of women treated for breast cancer report receiving support from specialist nurses (SSRU 1994: 50). However, it is not just *specialist* nurses who provide support. It is the small gestures and the detail of interpersonal communication that are remembered in positive terms. Wadler, for example, reports 'A nurse, hearing what is going on, silently brings me a cup of coffee, a small gesture that is enormously comforting' (Wadler 1992: 36).

Understanding information needs: problems and potential

If the role of specialist nurses in information giving has not yet gained unequivocal acceptance, this may be because nurses' own knowledge base concerning information needs and modes of communication remains limited. Assumptions about client information needs in breast disease are only now being supported and modified by research. Simplistic and stereotypical assumptions about who needs what information and when can still control the agenda for women ostensibly involved in decision making. One breast care nurse in the SSRU study reported:

> The first cynical thing is that they [doctors] make a pretty instant judgment about how intelligent individual women are and how frank they're going to be with them... I'm not really trying to knock them saying this. What do you do in a five minute consultation with someone you've never met before? You have to make instant judgements and they may be wrong. So all women are equal but some are definitely more equal than others.
>
> (SSRU 1994: 17)

Stress on the importance of full information giving needs to be accompanied by a knowledge of effective communication methods and timing. Ley and Spelman (1967) showed that information recall for medical outpatients was poor; approximately 40 per cent of the information had been lost 80 minutes later. Cimprich (1992) provided evidence to show the effects of limitations of attention and recall in life-threatening situations. Information, therefore, has to be pertinent to women's needs. Luker *et al.* (1993, 1996), in a study of women with breast cancer, have identified priority information needs as information about the likelihood of cure of breast cancer, information about stage and spread of the disease and information about treatment options. Information about the side-effects of treatment and about sexual attractiveness, often identified as important in the nursing literature (Marks-Maran and Pope 1985), were of lower priority. Luker *et al.* conclude that 'survival issues were a predominant concern for women... at diagnosis and overloading individuals with general non specific information at this time may only serve to overwhelm and confuse' (p. 494). This suggests that it is indeed information about probabilities of survival, information that remains within the domain of the medical profession, that is perceived as most important by women themselves.

What do women want? Difficulties and constraints in eliciting treatment preferences

If information about probabilities of treatments resulting in acceptable outcomes remains the expertise of professionals, it is women who 'know' which treatment choices are more acceptable to them. Eliciting women's preferences is seen as the role of a skilled breast care nurse. The problematic nature of this process remains relatively ill explored, but complicating factors include the recognition that women's perceptions of their feelings and views prior to diagnosis or prior to experiencing treatment are not good indicators of women's emotions at a later date. Women's utilities change. Furthermore, the utilities of healthy professionals, men or women, are poor bases for assumptions concerning appropriate care for women suffering from breast cancer. Slevin *et al.* (1990) found that doctors and nurses were less likely to accept radical treatment such as chemotherapy with minimal chance of benefit than were cancer patients. The researchers note that, 'although doctors may have the facts and statistics available they inevitably make subjective judgements in recommending a particular treatment option to patients'. Earlier research by the same team had shown that 'assessments of patients' quality of life and their levels of anxiety and depression by doctors and nurses correlate poorly with those made by the patients themselves' (Slevin *et al.* 1988).

It is important, therefore, for nurses to have a critical awareness of the limitations of their own knowledge concerning women's preferences and the possible misconceptions and biases that may influence published nursing literature. Despite extensive concern about women's fears of the effects of treatment on sexuality and attractiveness in the nursing literature (Marks-Maran and Pope 1985) and in published accounts from some women, Luker's research shows that information about sexual attractiveness was the least important in a list of nine information needs. Twenty-one months after diagnosis, while information on the likelihood of cure remained top of the list of information needs, information concerning risk to the family of developing cancer had moved to second place; sexual attractiveness remained the bottom priority. The importance that women themselves place on their own family and caring roles is often revealed in their responses to cancer diagnoses: 'I immediately thought of my poor husband' (Fallowfield 1991).

Nurses' assumptions

Women's first responses to diagnosis may provide cues to facilitate women's own identification of treatment preferences. Such facilitation is problematic but potentially empowering. Nurses' own assumptions may, however, inhibit this process. Nursing literature suggests a widespread acceptance of the idea that the loss of a breast is associated with a loss of self-esteem and that the impact of mastectomy is devastating, resulting in a need to mourn and to 'adjust to an acceptable reality' (RCN 1994b).The importance of recognising the psychological impact of a change of body shape should not be denied, but an uncritical association between loss of breast and loss of self-esteem can reinforce stereotypical constructions of female identity. The concern with body image is also imbued with heterosexism. A 1985 text, for example, notes:

> Most girls go through a phase of allowing other girls to touch their breasts at some time during their sexual development. This would seem to be a normal practice which precedes a heterosexual relationship. Once she notices boys are interested in her shape, she will start to buy bras and clothes which will enhance what 'mother nature' has given her.
>
> (Marks-Maran and Pope 1985: 7)

An uncritical acceptance of limited conceptions of womanhood can lead to distressing attention from those hoping to offer support. Anderson records a woman's account of and comment on a conversation with a hospital chaplain. 'He asked me how I was coping with my loss of womanhood... There's more to womanhood than a breast' (Anderson 1986: 75). Concern with women's breasts may unwittingly reinforce acceptance of the power of a male gaze.

Breast care nurses' assumptions may also be unacknowledgedly racist. Breast prostheses (like elastoplasts) have been pink, and the availability of colour variations has rarely been a topic of discussion. As Fallowfield (1991) explores, an ageist construction of women's concerns and likely treatment choices can also deny choice and limit care.

Breast care nurses may also wish to explore their assumptions concerning women's caring roles. Assumptions about such roles can be varied within both nursing literature and sociology. Whereas functionalist views may emphasise the normality of such roles, feminist standpoints may portray caring as an activity framed by a patriarchal society and performed by an oppressed group. Accounts of women as carers in literature on breast care often present women's caring orientation as a problem. Fallowfield (1991), in a chapter on delay in seeking advice, notes that female health professionals, especially nurses, report breast lumps later and have larger tumours. The reasons for this are not explored. Other accounts of 'delay' record putting family first:

> I didn't say anything to anyone 'cause I had the family here and I thought oh, dear, this will spoil everyone's Christmas.
>
> (Fallowfield 1991: 35)

There is little rationality attributed to such concern for others. Women's caring orientation may be constructed as part of patriarchal oppression, but the classification of such behaviour as 'delay' and hence as a problem is itself patriarchal.

More positive constructions are possible. Concern for others as a first and main response to one's cancer, for example, can be a coping mechanism and a source of strength. It is common. Anderson quotes a woman's response to her cancer as 'I only worry about my young one' (Anderson 1986: 81). Concern for others can limit concern for self and help to maintain a secure sense of identity despite threats to the body and life itself.

Making their own decisions: do women benefit?

The assumption that women wish to be involved in decisions about their treatment is rarely questioned. The possible *therapeutic* as well as ethical and legal importance of facilitating informed choice in breast cancer care has been highlighted through research into psychosocial adjustment in breast care. Some studies have suggested that participating in choice of treatment may lead to a decline in psychological morbidity (Ashcroft *et al.* 1985, Morris and Royle 1988) and thus promote health. Fallowfield (1991) and Cotton (1995), however, have noted the complexity of women's responses and the possibility of negative psychosocial effects. Encouraging women to share responsibility for treatment decisions may lead to psychological difficulties if the treatment choice is subsequently perceived as inappropriate. Cotton (1995) found that 5 out of 20 women in her 12-month follow-up study were *not* glad to have had a say in choice of treatment. It is by no means clear that all women wish to choose their own treatment. Research concerning the views of women treated for breast cancer, of women who have attended for mammographic screening and of professionals shows a preference for shared decision making, women deciding *with* their doctor (SSRU 1994). Promoting choice for women raises issues concerning women's right *not* to make their own decision. Some patients may prefer benevolent paternalism and seek a dependent role in the professional–client relationship, as the following comment illustrates:

> When he asked me what I wanted him to do I was very upset. I mean he's meant to be the expert isn't he? How should I be expected to know what's the best if he doesn't. I thought it was cruel.
>
> (Fallowfield 1991: 116)

Hidden agendas: participation in research

Involving clients in decision making, however, has sought to minimise the possible disadvantages of a paternalist professionalism. One of the possible disadvantages could be participation in clinical research without knowledge or consent. In the past, patients have been recruited into research studies that have contributed to the current knowledge base that informs breast cancer care. Hitherto, women were often recruited into studies without their knowledge. Now women may be asked to choose whether or not they are willing to enter a research trial. Although women may recognise and support the importance of research into breast cancer, the fact that their own participation in research into breast cancer treatment may be one of their options to consider is beyond the control of individual women, as is the availability of specialist expertise and resources. For women to make an informed choice about participating in research (a very different decision from supporting research in other ways), they need to understand the meaning of key terms such as 'randomisation', 'double blind' and 'randomised controlled trial'. Women's lack of understanding of the terms professionals take for granted can inhibit informed participation in decision making. The SSRU study found that almost half the women attending for breast cancer screening 'hadn't a clue' about the meaning of the terms 'control group' or 'randomisation', indicating the importance of information and clarification if women are to be asked to make decisions concerning participation in clinical trails. Such a request is common in breast cancer care (SSRU 1994: 122–3).

In consenting to participation in research, women are being asked to accept that professionals who are treating them do not know what is best for them as individuals and that their personal involvement in research may benefit future women who have the disease. Although altruism was the main reason given by women for agreeing to take part in research, the SSRU study found that three-fifths of women treated for breast cancer could not accept being randomised. They wanted to be able to choose treatment that was 'best' for them and would not exchange choice for chance. Medical uncertainty can be difficult to accept.

In being asked to facilitate women's informed consent to treatment trials, nurses themselves should understand the principle of equipoise, which assumes an honest belief that chances are equal and that no arm in the trial would be more likely to benefit a particular patient than another. If a professional believes that an option would be 'best' for one individual, it would not be ethical to ask that woman to enrol in a trial. In ascertaining what would be 'best' for an individual, we search for knowledge that is not just about statistical probabilities concerning probable survival rates, but is also additional personal knowledge about individual women's preferences and beliefs. If a nurse identifies that a woman has a particularly pessimistic view of survival rates after lumpectomy, for example, based on vivid personal recollections of a friend's disease, a nurse may be reluctant to recommend enrolling in a trial that may result in such treatment after randomisation. A nurse's 'hunch' that pessimism about a form of treatment may have negative psychological outcomes for a woman may not be seen as relevant information to a researcher who measures outcomes solely through survival rates. Nor may it be seen as legitimate information by other members of the health care team. A breast care nurse in the SSRU study eloquently explored her 'dis-ease' that derived from tensions in reconciling the personal impact of randomisation for individual women with broader responsibilities:

> At one end is Science, represented by the medical researchers and funders. They want to recruit large numbers into clinical trials to try to define once and for all, the most effective treatment for breast cancer...
>
> Since patient involvement in treatment choice became a publicly political issue and informed consent a prerequisite for ethical committee approval, women have been more likely to refuse to enter trials... So, Science needs an ethical way of persuading women to enter trials in large numbers...
>
> On the other pole... are the here-and-now breast cancer patients and their perceived information needs. They are grappling with the diagnosis of a life-threatening disease, making bizarre choices among previously unthinkably horrifying treatment alternatives, desperately looking for a lifeboat on a tilting deck when all the previously secure 'furniture' of their lives – relationships, career, responsibilities, finances, families – is hurtling past into the sea. No wonder randomisation, with its attendant depersonalisation is such a problem for women who feel threatened by the loss of their intrinsic selves anyway...
>
> I believe the better informed a woman is and the more good counselling and support she has, the less likely she is to agree to enter a trial. So much is already known... that it is hardly possible for many patients not to process this information... and to come up with an individually tailored package for themselves. (pp. 149–50)

Challenging knowledge

The analysis above identifies the significance of the movement towards involving clients in decision making. It is a challenge to accepted views about knowledge itself. Science shows itself to be uncertain; expert knowledge is incomplete. Doctors cannot easily recruit to clinical trials under the obligations of informed consent. The quote above does not acknowledge what other breast care nurses have identified: the medical profession needs nurses to facilitate recruitment to clinical trials in order to continue their approach to gathering knowledge and reducing their uncertainty. However, as the quotation does make clear, there are other sources of knowledge, sufficient, it is suggested, for women or professionals to make a judgement about what would be the best outcome for themselves *as individuals*. As Alderson points out in the SSRU report, '"best" has different meanings, ranging from *individually* appropriate to the patient, taking account of her hopes, fears and preferences, to *statistically* demonstrated to offer the best chance of a good outcome' (p. 150). There may be gender differences in the types of information valued and the way in which men and women use information. Riska and Wegar (1993) note that there is some evidence that women's style of communicating may allow psychosocial aspects to be identified (Meeuwesen *et al.* 1991). Additionally, there may be differences in a research orientation and a professional orientation. Although both doctors and nurses share ideals of individually planned care, medical clinicians are more likely to be familiar with and supportive of research orientations than are nurses. Women themselves have challenged the appropriateness of large-scale clinical trials (Thornton 1993).

Care-as-gift

Women make their own treatment choices through identifying what is important to them. In attempting to facilitate choice, nurses need to listen to women without prior assumptions about what they will or should want. In my practice as a breast care nurse, I found my 'academic' (sociological) interest in women's stories and in lay interpretations of health and disease to be an entirely natural adjuvant to my care. Listening to women's own framing of events facilitates links between lay and medical framing that may assist communication and decision making. Fox (1993) argues that nurses can foster a process of care that becomes an enabling 'care-as-gift'. In this perspective, the objective of care is 'to do with becoming and possibilities, about resistance to discourse, and a generosity towards otherness'. Such an approach seeks to avoid what Fox has termed 'care-as-discipline', an approach that constrains the cared-for within discourses that construct responses rather than enable individual expression. Assuming that women will be 'mourning loss of womanhood' can be seen as an example of 'care-as-discipline'. In the face of the evident uncertainty that breast cancer brings to professionals and clients, nurses seek to support women in taking control of their lives. How to do this is not and may never be clear, but, at the very least, nurses can seek to demonstrate a 'generosity towards otherness' that may allow women to react to a life-threatening disease in their own way, enabling women to identify their own feelings and their own hopes and fears. If, as Fox argues, 'care-as-gift' can be empowering, breast care nurses may thus enable women with breast disease to make their own decisions.

14 Caring for people with learning disabilities

Matthew Godsell

This chapter looks at advocacy and empowerment in the context of caring for people with learning disabilities. Analyses of power in nursing relationships, the influence of social policy and the impact of a wide range of social factors will be used to delineate issues that are pertinent to nurses and other carers involved in the delivery of services.

The focus of the chapter will be, first, the changing relationship between the social context in which care is delivered and the delivery of care, specifically the development of specialised residential services and their impact on the concepts, labels and the social construction of learning disabilities. Second, the chapter will focus on the role of nurses in the delivery of services and the exchange of power in the relationships that develop between service providers and service users.

Throughout the chapter, a socio-historic approach is used to make links between the current services and services in the past. By making connections between the present and the past, a different perspective emerges that places any evaluation of contemporary services against a historical background of continuity and change. Viewed from this perspective, it is increasingly difficult to regard the images, labels and stereotypes associated with different generations as a specific response to their particular characteristics or social situations. Each generation incorporates and builds on the images and symbols associated with preceding generations. Although a series of changes in social policy culminating in the NHS and Community Care Act 1990 have transformed service delivery, many of the images that surround people with learning disabilities reflect the experiences of other generations who spent their lives in workhouses, asylums or long-stay hospitals.

Whenever people with learning disabilities, nurses or carers attempt to change the negative images that surround them, they are often struggling to change an impression that has been left by history. The resistance they encounter is generated by this historical legacy as well as their current circumstances. In addition to the images and symbols that have been described, there are social, economic and political factors that run through historical periods and form direct links between the past and the present. The combination of factors discussed in this chapter suggest that it is too simplistic to attribute the qualitative differences that separate people with learning disabilities from other sectors of the population to institutionalisation or medicalisation. Although they have certainly been contributory factors, they can be located in larger schema in which the long-term influence of poverty, class, status and employment assume greater significance.

Historical information derived from public records frequently conveys information about the services that people have received without conveying significant details about the people who received them. Evidence from the late eighteenth and early nineteenth centuries has provided information about various attempts to assess the number of people with a learning disability. During 1881 a census return of 'idiots' in public institutions totalled 29,452 (Jones 1972: 182). In 1882 Daniel Hack Tuke stated that this figure was unreliable because it did not include a significant number of people who were unknown to the public authorities. Jones attributes inaccuracies like this to the 'submerged nature of the whole problem' (1972: 184). Figures that were derived from the number of people in public institutions would not reveal those who lived on their own, people living with their families or with other families. Data collected in public institutions would also exclude those people who were accommodated in private facilities. Sutherland (1984: 14) describes private madhouses as a 'well-established phenomena' by the late eighteenth century. Both comments suggest that a significant number of people have been ignored or excluded from any figures that were collected.

Inaccurate information about the number of people involved, together with a lack of understanding about where and how they lived, has led to the emergence of a succession of stereotypes, labels and myths. The images and beliefs that emerged focused on specific attributes of their lives. They encouraged people to overlook individual differences and pay less attention to the wide range of familial and social circumstances in which people lived.

Instead of portraying a variety of individual strengths and needs and an acknowledgement of different living arrangements, they depicted a limited number of characteristics that encouraged the more widespread presumption that these characteristics were indicative of everyone with a learning disability. These images tended to disregard the links that people with learning disabilities had with their local communities, families or friends. They also undermined their capacity for achievement by emphasising their reliance on public provision, philanthropy or charity as well as their need for care and supervision. The tenacity of these images continues to shape the public's perception despite more recent evidence that contradicts it.

The development of community care and the decline of large institutions has increased contact between those people who would have been 'patients' and the population outside the hospital. Although people with learning disabilities have a stronger presence in the community, they are still surrounded by images and ideas that connect them to a history of segregation and isolation in asylums and long-stay hospitals that stretches back to the Victorian era. Residence in a hospital has been synonymous with being 'locked up' or 'taken away'. The long association between learning disabilities and hospitalisation has remained in peoples' minds, while memories of other lifestyles and patterns of care have been relegated to the small groups of families or carers that sustained them. Hack Tuke pointed out that figures from the returns of 1881 were representative only of the number of people receiving a public service rather than the number of people with a learning disability. Brown, in the 1990s, points to a similar flaw in the figures relating to residential provision in the 1970s:

> The bulk of care is, and has always been, provided by informal carers, especially parents and in particular mothers. Precise figures are difficult to obtain. One commentary published by the Office of Health Economics estimated that in 1978 only one in every five individuals with severe mental handicap were living in residential provision. Four in every five individuals were being cared for at home. The historical emphasis upon residential services rather than upon where the bulk of care is carried out is very much a legacy of the Victorian era when care was equated with 'bricks and mortar' and the large institution.
>
> (1992: 107)

Both Brown and Hack Tuke suggest that the association between institutions and people with learning disabilities was forged in a discrete historical period and is not an accurate image of the way, or ways, in which a majority of people have received care.

The historical emphasis that has been placed on the 'bricks and mortar' of Victorian institutions has created a distorted image of the past. Accounts of the development and decline of institutionalisation have overshadowed other histories that describe alternative ways of delivering care and support outside the infrastructure of hospitals and workhouses. The impressions that have been left by these accounts are a testimony to the supremacy of a set of ideas and values that have dominated the decision making processes that underlie policy and regulation. These ideas are embedded in the collected voices of the professionals – the doctors, managers, administrators and nurses who have delivered health and welfare services. Their voices have overpowered the disparate voices of parents, carers and the users of the services. Their ability to create and control policy and provision indicates their capacity to wield power on three distinct levels.

Lukes' representation of the faces of power (1974) offers three different perspectives on the relationships between professionals and the laity (see Chapter 1). The first face of power has enabled professionals overtly to manipulate decision making so that they are able to promote their own interests above and beyond those of any other group or individual. While the first face has allowed them to bring together the resources, beliefs and values necessary to sustain their position, the second face of power has enabled them to exclude any opposing views or interests by placing restrictions or impediments around different aspects of the decision making process. The management, administration and regulation of a national system of institutions created a bureaucratic framework that gave a burgeoning class of professionals the power to impose their decisions on residents and their families. This was combined with the authority to control access to advisory boards and committees. The combination of these factors gave professionals control over the development of services at the expense of their users.

The third face of power has enabled the ideas perpetrated by this group to shape the attitudes and beliefs of the service users and their parents as well as the public's perception of both the services and the people associated with them. Such beliefs included their expectations regarding the role and function of the staff who worked in institutions in addition to the people who lived there. Institutions, and the specialised care provided by doctors and nurses, rather than life in the community shared with families or other carers, was the focus of policy and legislation. The administrative framework that was developed to regulate and monitor institutional provision reinforced particular roles and values that became established as the *status quo*. Means and Smith (1994) provide a useful summary of the history of neglect associated with the care of people with learning difficulties.

Policies that made explicit statements about the aims of services, and the production of documents and conceptual frameworks that measured the conduct of staff and residents, directed people's attention to a particular collection of norms and values (Ryan and Thomas 1980, Wright and Digby 1996). Because these ideas seemed to have the endorsement of the government and the support of those organised groups of people who were acknowledged as experts in the field, they dominated current thinking. Presenting opposing or alternative views would have entailed active participation in the policy process and a capacity to appeal to an alternative set of ideas or a different knowledge base. Organised groups of professionals were able to use their pre-eminent position to exercise the three faces of power so that parents of children with learning disabilities, adults with learning disabilities and the general public were excluded from participation at this level.

Professional dominance has not been confined to the developmental stages of services. It was a integral part of institutions and still continues to exert a powerful influence on service delivery in the present. Professionals were regarded as a legitimate target for criticism by the Conservative government in the 1980s:

> From its inception, professionals were an integral element in the wide range of services encompassing the welfare state. Increasingly, during the 1980s they were depicted as part of the non-productive public sector, a powerful constraint on change, acting more in their own interests than those of their clients and supporters of big government.
>
> (Gladstone 1995: 19)

During this period, the extent of the power they had wielded in the health services was questioned.

Thomson (1992) has discerned two separate aspects of community care that have been influential in determining service provision following the inter-war period. Both of the aspects that he described impinge on the development of roles for the people who use the services and the professionals who deliver them. He identified a 'fundamental ambiguity' in community care that has its origins in the 1913 Mental Deficiency Act. The Act set out to ensure 'that care should be provided to protect the defective from the community, yet also to protect the community from the defective' (Thomson 1992: 6).

These two aspects of service provision have had repercussions on the ways in which service users and providers have regarded themselves and the ways in which they have been perceived by other people. Measures that aimed to 'protect the community from the defective' clearly labelled the individual or the population of people with learning disabilities as dangerous or contagious (or both). Measures that aimed to 'protect the community from the defective' convey suspicion and mistrust about the communities from which those individuals came. Thomson argued that this mistrust pervaded the reports of visitors to working-class homes. He has also stated that the general lack of sympathy for indigenous community care has meant that supervision within the community has been seen as 'a second best alternative rather than a replacement of community care' (1992: 6). Both of these attributes have contributed to the stock of images and ideas associated with nurses working with people with learning disabilities.

Practitioners working in current services are encouraged to regard advocacy and empowerment as key elements in their work. Although the nursing curriculum has made them important aspects of the nurse's role, the contemporary nurse is also surrounded by a host of historical images that incorporate those mentioned by Thomson. These images have imbued professionals with the attributes that he has described. On the one hand, they have been charged with safeguarding the welfare of the community by protecting it from the contagion of mental deficiency. On the other hand, they have also been given the responsibility for protecting and defending the same group of people from any external threats. They were expected to use their training and status to act as guardians and protect any defectives in their care from exploitation, abuse and ignorance within their indigenous community. Newspaper reporting of incidents around The Walled Garden, a community home in Calcot near Reading, provides evidence suggesting that these images have retained some credence in the 1990s. The report describes how some of the established residents have responded to their neighbours with learning disabilities:

> I can't explain the noises they make. It's like an animal noise and it's not only day, it's night as well. I'm ashamed of (Virginia) Bottomley. She ought to be shot.

The 53-year-old woman was furious. She would not be named but was adamant that the small private road near Calcot golf club was 'not the right place for these people' (Jury 1993: 3).

The speaker has separated the residents of The Walled Garden from the rest of the village in two distinct ways. They are seen as possessing characteristics and behaviours that are not compatible with those of their neighbours. The way in which they conduct their lives and the noises they produce appear to be beyond explanation, resembling the nocturnal behaviour of animals rather than humans. Her description suggests that she regards the presence of people with learning disabilities as a blight on her community; Calcot is not seen as an appropriate place for them to live. Alternatives have not been provided, but the suggestion that their behaviour is not suited to the rhythms and routines of village life indicates that this lady may have found the secure and secluded environment of an institution a more acceptable proposition.

Another interviewee continued to make analogies between the residents and animals. In the following description, the noises they produce are likened to foxes and an animal being killed:

> The noise they make frightens the children. The first time I thought it was an animal being killed or something. I rushed out. After a while you get used to it. You know it is them. We've got foxes and everything in the lane, but you realise now when it's a patient.
>
> (Jury 1993: 3)

In addition to making noises like animals and disrupting the villagers' quiet lives, they are also seen as a potential threat. The residents evoke a fearful response in the local children. Reference to an animal being killed creates an especially sinister context for the delivery of this remark. The speaker ends by making an explicit reference to 'patients'. Although the residents no longer live in a hospital, this description has followed them to their new home. It may have been intended as a factual description of their former residence, but it can also be interpreted as a statement expressing the speaker's views on the most appropriate type of residence for them.

The newspaper report has accentuated the ways in which local residents have perceived differences between their own lifestyles, values and behaviour and those they have attributed to their neighbours from The Walled Garden. People with learning disabilities are perceived as a potential threat to the social fabric of the village as well as causing the destruction of a tranquil idyll that had prevailed prior to their arrival. In addition to the immediate problem caused by noise, there is the more pervasive threat that hangs over the future of the village. It concerns what may happen rather than what is actually happening. There is a suggestion that if the residents are permitted to remain in The Walled Garden, the quality of life for the rest of the villagers must deteriorate. The view that the presence of people with a learning disability will lead to an overall decline in the standards also has a historical precedent:

> Let us assume that we could segregate as a community all the families in this country containing mental defectives of the primary amentia type. We would find that we had collected among them a most interesting social group. It would include, as everyone who has extensive practical experience of social service would readily admit, a much larger proportion of insane persons, epileptics, paupers, criminals (especially recidivists), unemployable, habitual slum dwellers, prostitutes, inebriates and other social inefficients than would a group of families not containing mental defectives. The overwhelming majority of the families thus collected will belong to the community which we propose to term the 'social problem' or 'subnormal group'.
>
> (Ryan and Thomas 1980: 108)

The report has suggested that the behaviour and morals of mentally defective people constitute a 'social problem' for other sections of society. In addition to degrading the environment by creating and perpetuating slum dwellings, they have also threatened the moral fabric of society through pauperism, criminal behaviour, prostitution and inebriation. The Board of Control used this as a rationale for implementing measures that would control and contain the population by segregation and a prohibition on marriage. The implementation of these measures was seen as a way of protecting the nation from 'the racial disaster of mental deficiency' (Ryan and Thomas 1980: 108). It is in this context that institutions emerged as a way of imposing a *cordon sanitaire* around people with learning disabilities, and the staff working with them acquired the roles of guardians and custodians.

The people who were described by the Board of Control and the residents of The Walled Garden share a similar position. They have been pushed out to the margins of society, where they occupy a moral and geographical space that has been separated from the rest of the community. The newspaper reports do not feature any quotations from the staff or the residents. Other peoples' descriptions have accentuated the former's need to provide supervision and the latter's need to receive it. The reports hint at both the vulnerability and volatility of people with learning disabilities. The role of custodian or guardian is not consistent with the roles of citizen, facilitator and advocate that are emerging from the current nursing curriculum. In these roles, nurses are directed to improve integration by enhancing the capacity of services and individuals to assert their presence in the community and maintain a level of active participation (O'Brien 1981).

As services have moved out of hospitals into the community, both staff and residents have had to contend with the legacy of the past. Residential settings in villages, towns and city streets have created more opportunities for mixing with other people who are carrying out everyday activities. At the same time, those opportunities have also brought them face to face with the public's prejudice, fear and suspicion. Carers and clients may have to confront angry neighbours or abusive children in situations that would not have occurred in an isolated, institutional setting. As the services have moved from hospitals into the community, staff have had to take on roles as mediators and advocates. They may find themselves presenting the case for empowerment to a sceptical public who believe that the best place for a person with a learning disability is in a hospital. In this capacity, they have had to acquire different skills that enable them to work in liaison with the public as well as clients. To achieve this, they have had to abandon the security of their former status as 'detached' professionals who conducted their work in isolation. Nurses working with people with learning disabilities will also be cognisant of an ideological shift in their power base. Individualised care in this social context entails sharing power with clients and responding to their needs, desires, wishes and opinions. Power and authority are derived from a nurses' capacity to work co-operatively *with* clients rather than imposing their own ideas on them.

As nurses have moved away from institutional settings, their role within services has undergone a series of transformations. Although many nurses now work in community homes rather than hospitals, they still have responsibility for maintaining the environment in which their clients live. Hospitals had a discrete administrative and managerial structure that diverted some of the responsibility for paperwork, budgets, provisions, cleaning and cooking away from them. Nurses working in community homes have found that they need to devote much of their time to these matters, particularly their responsibilities regarding budgeting and administration. While their commitment to creating more choices and encouraging participation aligns them with clients, their other responsibilities can distort their role as an advocate. Working alongside clients makes them conscious of their social, educational and recreational needs as well as the resources that are required to satisfy them. At the same time, their employers will remind them of restraints on spending and reinforce their obligation to remain within their allocated budget. Nurses are divided between their conflicting roles as advocates and managers.

In some instances, nurses advocating on behalf of clients may be accused of reinforcing their professional status and the dependent image of people with learning disabilities. A significant proportion of people with learning disabilities rely on carers or professionals to articulate the case for maintaining or developing services. Unlike other minority groups who have developed political strategies or organised pressure groups to instigate changes in policy and provision, they lack the power and resources to make themselves heard. This contributes to the social construction of their disability by creating the impression of a double disadvantage. They lack the power and status conferred by wealth, as well as the mechanisms to generate political organisation or collective action that would enable them to present their oppression as a social issue. Where professional groups or charities take on this role, they can be accused of implementing their own agendas or depriving people with learning disabilities of an opportunity to assert themselves.

Nurses working with people with learning disabilities form a link between the past and the future. Although the social roles occupied by both nurses and people with learning disabilities are changing, there are persistent reminders of the past. Advocacy and empowerment provide nurses with a philosophy for transforming the delivery of services, but their capacity to effect any radical change is limited by the conservative nature of their former roles and the obligations that divide their loyalties. The division between health and social care may also divert nurses from a concerted drive towards political and social change.

The development of community care and the polarisation of health and social care have altered the ways in which services for people with learning disabilities are delivered. While these services have been undergoing revision, nursing has also been influenced by changes that have reverberated through all of its branches. These changes have transformed both education and practice. The status of nurses, their credibility as professionals and the impact that status may have on their relationships with patients, clients and service users have been critically evaluated. Some nurses seem to relish the prospect of increasing professional status. Others regard it as an impediment to the advancement of working relationships with clients and colleagues that could be closer and more open. While some would see professional knowledge, autonomy and self-management as axiomatic for the progress of nursing, Davies has described the detrimental effects they can have on teamwork:

> The classic professional, because of superior knowledge, will claim autonomy and self-management, arguing that practice cannot be regulated by those who are not versed in the requisite knowledge bases. Each professional must be self-regulating and peer review is the only appropriate form of monitoring. The corollary of all this is that the professional bears a heavy weight of responsibility for decisions made.
>
> Such a burden serves further to separate the professional from others, and indeed nurses often report that they will defer to the doctor because in the end the doctor carries the can. However, here too is the beginning of a shift in the emphasis with preceptorship and mentoring and also clinical supervision. Individual responsibility for maintaining and developing standards gives way, for less rigidly bounded individuals, to an

> acceptance that care is a team phenomenon, and drawing out and enhancing the contributions others, whatever their formal roles and titles, can be beneficial. This raises the challenge of how a collective can be held to account if boundaries between professions and between professionals and non-professionals remain as strong as they are today.
> (1996: 54)

The article describes a departure from the established conception of professional practice and a movement towards a more collective approach. This way of working involves the abandonment of any former notions of detachment and élitism as well as cultivating the capacity to work with a mixture of people in a variety of roles.

The changes that have occurred in and around services for people with learning disabilities have encouraged the nurses working in them to utilise some of the characteristics that Davies has described. The adoption of the individual programme planning process (Phoenix NHS Trust and Avon Social Services 1995) has pointed to the need to foster services that are more responsive to the needs of service users. To continue developing along these lines, practitioners need to form co-operative working arrangements with clients. In these circumstances, nurses cannot maintain a professional aloofness that separates them from everybody else. Nor can they preserve rigid boundaries around individual responsibility based on their claims to autonomy and self-management. Working as a collective may involve sharing responsibilities with other members of the care team, but if services are going to become 'client centred', decision making has to include clients and their families or advocates.

In addition to the changes that have transformed their relationships with service users, learning disability nurses working in the community are also having to adjust to a higher public profile. Their activities and the decisions that they make are more visible than they have ever been before. Nurses deliver care alongside clients who are based in the community rather than isolated behind the closed doors of a hospital ward. Living and working in the community entails a degree of responsibility towards the other people who live there. Although nurses may need the support and guidance of their peers, they are also accountable to the people they meet everyday as fellow citizens, voters, consumers of public services and neighbours.

Conclusion

This book has explored power issues in nursing practice. It has found power embedded in aspects of social structures, made visible through managerial and professional hierarchies, through the mechanisms of the labour market and the division of labour in health care, through health policies and through the organisation of care. Cultural assumptions about gender, age and education, and limited public discourse about the intimacy of care all influence nurses' and clients' power and authority. Power is at work in relationships between nurses and clients, nurses and nurses, nurses and other professional groups. Whereas power is made visible through decision making, agenda setting, communication and interaction styles, it is also hidden in the taken-for-granted and is only noticed through the careful observation of change. Differences in the use of physical space, differences in posture and in the non-verbal communication of a sense of trust, differences in discourse have all been noted as indicative of the possibilities of nursing power.

Power issues in nursing will be most effectively explored by nurses themselves when they have the confidence to analyse power from a range of theoretical standpoints and the confidence to seek to effect change. Sociology teaches us that it is possible to argue that where there is power there is resistance, and where there is action, there is the chance to make a difference. Discourses can be shaped and used. The power of support and care can be explored. Sociology also teaches us that such exploration is best framed by a realistic appraisal of the power of élites, hierarchies, organisations, patriarchal cultures and inequalities associated with class, gender, age, race, ethnicity, sexuality and disability.

In exploring power issues, however, authors have not necessarily confined themselves to drawing on sociological theories. Whereas Miers' and Wilkinson's chapters make explicit use of sociological approaches, other authors have made use of a more eclectic range of literature, drawing on social policy, on feminist literature and on nursing's own analysis. This is perhaps an interesting reminder to sociologists that what practitioners need are the intellectual and empirical tools to analyse the social context of nursing and how it affects their practice. The disciplinary origins of these tools are not necessarily the practitioner's concern. It is not just sociology that illuminates the social dimensions of nursing care. It is hoped that the chapters' varied approaches in themselves provide an opportunity for readers to reflect on how different approaches highlight or observe power issues in practice.

Whereas all the authors have been concerned to identify the importance of the social context for an understanding of power, few have directly explored how a sociological understanding of power might enhance nursing practice. The use of sociological theory in a practice discipline is a challenge that few nurses or sociologists explicitly address. Morrall (1996), however, has argued that sociological theories can demystify power and argues that planned positive social change is possible on an individual casework basis. His view is that sociology could provide a basis for therapeutic action in mental health. These are bold claims, neither explored nor supported here; nevertheless, this series is committed to opening up debate about the importance of sociologically informed nurses and sociologically informed nursing care.

The challenge is for both nurses and sociologists to develop relationships that are fruitful and productive both for themselves and, most importantly, for those who use health and welfare services. This may require nurses to open up to others about the nature of the work they do and the demands that it makes; for sociologists, the task is in accessing a hitherto hidden world and finding ways of revealing it that demeans none of the participants. The task may involve a reflexive analysis of one's own use of power and a critique of one's own praxis. The reward lies in recognising the joint nature of the project and valuing the potential positive outcomes for all involved in the provision of health and social care.

References

Abbott P and Wallace C (1990a) *An Introduction to Sociology: Feminist Perspectives*. Routledge, London.

Abbott P and Wallace C (1990b) The sociology of the caring professions: an introduction. In Abbott P and Wallace C (eds) *The Sociology of the Caring Professions*. Falmer, London, pp. 1–9.

Abel Smith B (1968) *A History of the Nursing Profession*. Heinemann, London.

Acker J (1990) Hierarchies, jobs and bodies: a theory of gendered organisations. *Gender and Society* **4**: 139–58.

Acker J (1991) Hierarchies, jobs and bodies: a theory of gendered organisation. In Lorber J and Farrell S (eds) *The Social Construction of Gender.* Sage, London, pp. 162–79.

Ackroyd S (1993) Towards an understanding of nurses' attachments to their work. *Journal of Advances in Health and Nursing Care* **2**(3): 23–46.

Ackroyd S (1995) Nurses, management and morale: a diagnosis of decline in the NHS hospital service. In Soothill K, McKay L and Webb C (eds) *Interprofessional Relations in Health Care*. Edward Arnold, London, pp. 222–38.

Age Concern England (1993) *Moving the Goalposts*. Age Concern England, London.

Air M (1996) Scottish Breast Cancer campaign. *Breast Care Nursing* Summer: 3–4.

Allen D (1997) The nursing–medical boundary: a negotiated order? *Sociology of Health and Illness* **19**(4): 498–520.

Allmark P and Klarzynski R (1992) The case against nurse advocacy. *British Journal of Nursing* **2**(1): 33–6.

Althusser L (1970) *Ideology and Ideological State Apparatuses (Notes toward an investigation)*. Verso, London.

Anderson M J (1986) *The Nursing Contribution to the Aftercare of the Mastectomy Patient*. Department of Nursing Studies, University of Edinburgh.

Armstrong D (1983) *Political Anatomy of the Body: Medical Knowledge in Britain in the Twentieth Century*. Cambridge University Press, Cambridge.

Ashcroft J J, Leinster S J and Slade P D (1985) Breast cancer: patient choice of treatment. *Journal of the Royal Society of Medicine* **78**: 43.

Ashworth P (1990) High technology and humanity for intensive care. *Intensive Care Nursing* **6**(3): 150–60.

Atkinson J (1986) *Changing Work Patterns: How Companies Achieve Flexibility to Meet New Needs*. National Economic Development Office, London.

Atkinson P (1977) Professional segmentation and students' experience in a Scottish medical school. *Scottish Journal of Sociology* **2**: 71–85.

Atkinson P (1981) Bernstein's structuralism. *Educational Analysis* **3**: 85–96.

Audit Commission (1991) *The Virtue of Patients: Making Best Use of Ward Nursing Resources*. HMSO, London.

Aust R, Boddy G and Newall J (1996) *Nurses' Use of Sociological Concepts*. Paper presented at the RCN Research Society Conference, Newcastle, March 1996.

Aust R, Fraher A, Limpinnian M *et al.* (1997) *Power, Policy and Practice*. Faculty of Health and Social Care, University of the West of England, Bristol.

Bachrach P and Baratz M S (1962) Two faces of power. *American Political Science Review* **56**: 542–7.

Baker P (1997) A practical way forward in forging alliances. *Nursing Times* **93**(27): 42.

Barber B (1963) Some problems in the sociology of the professions. *Daedalus* **92**(4): 669–88.

Barker I, Maines K and Wright L (1993) Consumers voices in purchasing. In Beresford P and Harding T (eds) *A Challenge to Change: Practical Experience of Building User-led Services*. National Institute for Social Work, London.

Barker P (1993) *Michel Foucault: Subversions of the Subject*. Harvester Wheatsheaf, Hemel Hempstead.

Barker P J (1997) *Assessment in Psychiatric and Mental Health Nursing*. Stanley Thornes, Cheltenham.

Baron S and Haldane J (eds) (1992) *Community, Normality and Difference: Meeting Social Needs*. Aberdeen University Press, Aberdeen.

Barrett M (1980) *Women's Oppression Today*. Verso, London.

Barrett M and McIntosh M C (1991) *The Anti Social Family*, 2nd edn. Verso, London.

Barron R D and Norris G M (1976) Sexual divisions and the dual labour market. In Barker D L and Allen S (eds) *Dependence and Exploitation in Work and Marriage*. Longman, London.

Beardshaw V and Robinson R (1990) *New for Old? Prospects for Nursing in the 1990s*. King's Fund Institute, London.

Beattie A (1995) War and peace among the health tribes. In Soothill K, Mackay L and Webb C (eds) *Interprofessional Relations in Health Care*. Edward Arnold, London, pp. 11–26.

Becker H, Geer B, Hughes E and Strauss A (1961) *Boys in White*. University of Chicago Press, Chicago.

Benner P (1984) *From Novice to Expert: Excellence and Power in Clinical Nursing*. Addison-Wesley, Menlo Park, CA.

Beresford P (1993) Current issues in user involvement and empowerment. In Beresford P and Harding T (eds) *A Challenge to Change: Practical Experience of Building User-led Services*. National Institute for Social Work, London.

Best S and Kellner D (1991) *Postmodern Theory – Critical Interrogation*. Macmillan, Basingstoke.

Bidwell R J (1988) The gay and lesbian teen: a case of denied adolescence. *Journal of Paediatric Health Care* **2**(1): 3–8.
Biggs S (1993) *Understanding Ageing: Images, Attitudes and Professional Practice*. Open University Press, Buckingham.
Biley F (1992) Some determinants that effect patient participation in decision-making about nursing care. *Journal of Advanced Nursing* **17**: 414–21.
Bloor M and McIntosh J (1990) Surveillance and concealment: a comparison of techniques of client resistance in therapeutic communities and health visiting. In Cunningham Burley S and McKeganey N (eds) *Readings in Medical Sociology*. Routledge, London, pp. 159–81.
Bond J and Bond S (1994) *Sociology and Health Care*. Churchill Livingstone, Edinburgh.
Booth T (1993) Obstacles to the development of user centred services. In Johnson J and Slater R (eds) *Ageism and Later Life*. Sage, London, pp. 160–7.
Bowman M (1983) Nursing by lamplight. *Health Services* **46**: 10–11.
Brahams D (1985) Doctor's duty to inform patient of substantial or special risks when offering treatment. *Lancet* March 2: 528–30.
Braverman H (1974) *Labor and Monopoly Capitalism*. Monthly Review Press, New York.
Brown G (1993) Accounting for power: nurse teachers and students perceptions in their relationship. *Nurse Education Today* **13**: 111–20.
Brown J (1992) The residential setting in mental handicap: an overview of selected policy inititiatives 1971–89. In Thompson T and Mathias P (eds) *Standards and Mental Handicap: Keys to Competence*. Baillière Tindall, London.
Brown J S T and Furstenberg A (1992) Restoring control: empowering older patients and their families during health crisis. *Social Work Health Care* 17(4): 81–101.
Budge L, McKay D and Marsh D (1983) *The New British Political System*. Longman, London.
Bunton R (1990) Regulating our favourite drug. In Abbott P and Payne G (eds) *New Directions in the Sociology of Health*. Falmer Press, London.
Bytheway W and Johnson J (1990) On defining ageism. *Critical Social Policy* **10**(2): 27–39.
Caines K (1996) Here to there. *Nursing Standard* **10**(45): 18.
Calman K and Hine D (1995) *A Policy Framework for Cancer Commissioning*. DoH, London.
Campbell T and Heginbotham C (1991) *Mental Illness and Prejudice, Discrimination and the Law*. Aldershot, Dartmouth.
Carlile G (1996) Telling it like it is. *Nursing Times* **92**(11): 50–2.
Carpenter M (1993) The subordination of nurses in health care: towards a social divisions approach. In Riska E and Wegar K (eds) *Gender, Work and Medicine*. Sage, London, pp. 95–130.
Carr-Saunders A M and Wilson P A (1962) *The Professions*. Oxford University Press, London.

Carter H (1994) Confronting patriarchal attitudes in the fight for professional recognition. *Journal of Advanced Nursing* **19**(2): 367–72.
Cassell P (ed.) (1993) *The Giddens Reader*. Macmillan, Basingstoke.
Castel R (1991) From dangerousness to risk. In Burchell G, Gordon C and Miller P (eds) *The Foucault Effect: Studies in Governmentality*. Harvester Wheatsheaf, Brighton.
Central Statistical Office (1996) *Social Trends* 26. HMSO, London.
Charles N and Hughes-Freeland F C (1996) *Practising Feminism*. Routledge, London.
Cheek J and Rudge T (1994) The panoptican revisited?: an exploration of the social and political dimensions of contemporary health care and nursing practice. *International Journal of Nursing Studies* **31**(6): 583–91.
Cimprich B (1992) Attentional fatigue following breast cancer surgery. *Research in Nursing and Health* **15**: 199–207.
Collins P H (1990) *Black Feminist Thought: Knowledge, Consciousness and the Politics of Empowerment*. Routledge, London.
Connell R (1987) *Gender and Power*. Allen & Unwin, London.
Cotton T (1995) Patient choice in breast cancer treatment. *Nursing Times* **91**(17): 12.
Coward R (1990) *The Whole Truth*. Faber & Faber, London.
Crompton R (1987) Gender, status and professionalism. *Sociology* **21**(3): 413–28.
Dalley G (1988) *Ideologies of Caring – Rethinking Community and Collectivism*. Macmillan, Basingstoke.
Davies C (1980) *Rewriting Nursing History*. Croom Helm, London.
Davies C (1992) Gender, history and management style in nursing: towards a theoretical synthesis. In Witz A and Savage M (eds) *Gender and Bureaucracy*. Blackwell, Oxford.
Davies C (1995) *Gender and the Professional Predicament in Nursing*. Open University Press, Buckingham.
Davies C (1996a) The sociology of professions and the profession of gender. *Sociology* **30**(4): 661–78.
Davies C (1996b) A new vision of professionalism. *Nursing Times* **92**(46): 54–8.
Davies C and Francis A (1976) *Perceptions of Structure in NHS Hospitals*. Sociological Review Monograph 22. University of Keele, Staffordshire.
Davies C and Rosser J (1986) *Processes of Discrimination: A Study of Women Working in the NHS*. DHSS, London.
Davies J A, parent's reaction (audiocassette tape) Pitman Medical. Cited in Woodhouse S (1990) Why have medicine rounds? *Paediatric Nursing* **2**(10: 9–11.
Davis K (1991) Critical sociology and gender relations. In Davis K, Leijenaar M and Oldersma J (eds) *The Gender of Power*. Sage, London.
Deevey S (1990) Older lesbian women. An invisible minority. *Journal of Gerontological Nursing* **16**(5): 35–9.
Department of Health (1989) *Caring for People: Community Care in the Next Decade and Beyond*. HMSO, London.

Department of Health (1991) *The Patient's Charter*. DoH, London.
Department of Health (1992a) *The Health of the Nation*. DoH, London.
Department of Health (1992b) *The Children Act, a Training and Study Pack for NHS Personnel Workbook*. HMSO, London.
Department of Health (1993) *A Strategy for Nursing, Midwifery and Health Visiting Research*. DoH, London.
Department of Health (1994) *Working in Partnership: A Collaborative Approach to Care*. HMSO, London.
Department of Health (1995) *Non medical education and training – planning guidance for 1995/6 education commissioning*. NHS Executive, Leeds.
Department of Health (1997a) *The New NHS*. The Stationery Office, London.
Department of Health (1997b) *NHS The Patient's Charter: Mental Health Services*. DoH, London.
Department of Health and Social Security (1981) *Care in the Community: A Consultative Document in Moving Resources for Care in England*. DHSS, London.
Department of Health/Social Services Inspectorate (1991) *Care Management and Assessment: Summary of Practice Guidance*. HMSO, London.
Dingwall R and McIntosh M (eds) (1978) *Readings in the Sociology of Nursing*. Churchill Livingstone, Edinburgh.
Douglas M (1975) *Implicit Meanings: Essays in Anthropology*. Routledge & Kegan Paul, London.
Dowling S and Barrett S (1991) *Doctors in the Making: The Experiences of the Pre-registration Year*. University of Bristol, Bristol.
Doyal L, Hunt G and Mellor J (1981) Your life in their hands: migrant workers in the National Health Service. *Critical Social Policy* **1**(2): 54–71.
Durkheim E (1967) *The Division of Labour in Society*. Free Press, New York.
Dworkin A (1981) *Pornography: Men Possessing Women*. Women's Press, London.
Ehrenreich B and English D (1973) *Witches, Midwives and Nurses: A History of Women Healers*. London Compendium, London.
Eliason M J (1993) Cultural diversity in nursing care: the lesbian, gay or bisexual client. *Journal of Transcultural Nursing* **5**(1): 14–19.
Ellis K (1993) *Squaring the Circle: User Participation in Needs Assessment*. Joseph Rowntree Foundation in association with Community Care, York.
Ellis P (1992) Role of the nurse advocate. *British Journal of Nursing* **1**(1): 40–3.
Engels F (1972) *The Origin of The Family, Private Property and the State*. Lawrence & Wishart, London.
English National Board for Nursing, Midwifery and Health Visiting (1995) *The Contribution of Service Users and Carers to Education and Training*. ENB, London.

Etzioni A (1969) *The Semi-professions and their Organisation*. Free Press, New York.
Fairchild S K, Carrino G E and Ramirez M (1996) Social worker's perceptions of staff attitudes of ward residents' sexuality in a random sample of New York nursing homes; a pilot study. *Journal of Gerontological Social Work* **26**(1/2): 153–69.
Fallowfield L (1991) *Breast Cancer*. Routledge, London.
Farmer B (1993) The use and abuse of power in nursing. *Nursing Standard* 7(23): 33–6.
Fennell G, Phillipson C and Evers H (1988) *The Sociology of Old Age*. Open University Press, Buckingham.
Field D (1984) 'We didn't want him to die on his own' – nurses' accounts of nursing dying patients. *Journal of Advanced Nursing* **9**: 59–70.
Finch J and Groves D (1983) *Labour of Love*. Routledge & Kegan Paul, London.
Firestone S (1972) *The Dialectics of Sex*. Paladin, London.
Forgacs D (1988) *A Gramsci Reader*. Lawrence & Wishart, London.
Foucault M (1976) *The Birth of the Clinic: An Archaeology of Medical Perception*. Tavistock, London.
Foucault M (1978) *The History of Sexuality*. Penguin, Harmondsworth.
Foucault M (1979) *The History of Sexuality,* Vol. 1: *An Introduction*. Allen Lane, London.
Foucault M (1980) Power and knowledge. In Gordon C (ed.) *Selected Interviews and Other Writings*. Harvester Wheatsheaf, Brighton.
Foucault M (1982) Afterword: the subject and power. In Dreyfus H and Rabinow P (eds) *Michel Foucault: Beyond Structuralism and Hermeneutics*. University of Chicago Press, Chicago, pp. 208–26.
Foucault M (1991a [1975]) *Discipline and Punish: The Birth of the Prison*. Penguin Books, Harmondsworth.
Foucault M (1991b) Governmentality. In Burchell G, Gordon C and Miller P (eds) *The Foucault Effect*. Harvester Wheatsheaf, Brighton, pp. 53–72.
Fox N (1993) *Postmodernism, Sociology and Health*. Open University Press, Buckingham.
Freidson E (1970) *Profession of Medicine: A Study in the Sociology of Applied Knowledge*. Dodd Mead, New York.
Freidson E (1984) The changing nature of professional control. *Annual Review of Sociology* **10**: 1–20.
Freidson E (1994) *Professionalism Reborn: Theory, Prophecy and Policy*. Polity Press, Cambridge.
Freire P (1970) *Pedagogy of the Oppressed*. Seabury Press, New York.
Gamarnikow E (1978) Sexual division of labour: the case of nursing. In Kuhn A and Wolpe A (eds) *Feminism and Materialism*. Routledge & Kegan Paul, London, pp. 96–123.
Game A and Pringle R (1984) *Gender at Work*. Pluto, London.
Gerth H H and Mills C W (1948) *From Max Weber: Essays in Sociology*. Routledge & Kegan Paul, London.

Gibson C (1991) A concept analysis of empowerment. *Journal of Advanced Nursing* **16**: 354–61.
Giddens A (1971) *Capitalism and Modern Social Theory*. Cambridge University Press, Cambridge.
Giddens A (1984) *The Constitution of Society*. Polity Press, Cambridge.
Giddens A (1990) *The Consequences of Modernity*. Polity Press, Cambridge.
Gilbert L A (1993) *Two Careers, One Family: The Promise of Gender Equality*. Sage, London.
Gilligan C (1982) *In a Different Voice*. Harvard University Press, Cambridge, MA.
Gladstone D (1995) *British Social Welfare: Past, Present and Future*. University College, London Press, London.
Goddard H (1953) *The Work of Nurses in Hospital Wards. Report of a Job Analysis*. Nuffield Provincial Hospital Trust, Oxford.
Godden J, Curry G and Delacour S (1993) The decline of myths and myopia? The use of and abuse of nursing history. *Australian Journal of Advanced Nursing* **10**(2): 27–34.
Goffman E (1961) *Asylums*. Penguin, Harmondsworth.
Graham A (1992) Advocacy: what the future holds. *British Journal of Nursing* **1**(3): 148–50.
Graham H (1984) *Women, Health and the Family*. Harvester Wheatsheaf, Brighton.
Graham H (1993) *Hardship and Health in Womens' Lives*. Harvester Wheatsheaf, Brighton.
Gramsci A (1916) The popular university. In Forgacs D (1988) *A Gramsci Reader*. Lawrence & Wishart, London.
Gramsci A (1971) *Selections from the Prison Notebooks*. Lawrence & Wishart, London.
Gray P, Kramer M, Minick P, McGehee L, Thomas D, and Greiner D (1996) Heterosexism in nursing education. *Journal of Nursing Education* **35**(5): 204–10.
Greenwood E (1957) Attributes of a profession. *Social Work* **2**(3): 44–5.
Griffiths R (1983) *NHS Management Enquiry*. DHSS, London.
Guardian (1991) Time running out to avert elderly crisis. 30 Sept: 6.
Gwilliam C and Gilliard J (1996) Dementia and the social model of disability. *Journal of Dementia Care* **4**(1): 14–15.
Habenstein R W and Christ E A (1955) *Professionaliser, Traditionaliser and Utiliser*. University of Missouri, Columbia, MO.
Habermas J (1984) *The Theory of Communicative Action*, Vol. 1: *Reason and Rationalisation of Society*. Heinemann, London.
Hakim C (1979) *Occupational Segregation*. Department of Employment Research Papers 9. HMSO, London.
Hall J M (1994) Lesbians recovering from alcohol problems: an ethnographic study of health care experiences. *Nursing Research* **43**(4): 238–44.
Haralambos M and Holborn M (1991) *Sociology: Themes and Perspectives*, 3rd edn. Collins Educational, London.

Hartmann H (1976) Capitalism, patriarchy and job segregation by sex. In Giddens A and Held D (eds) *Classes, Power and Conflict – Classical and Contemporary Debates*. Macmillan, Basingstoke, pp. 446–69.
Hartmann H (1979) Capitalism, patriarch and job segregation by sex. In Esentein Z (ed.) *Capitalist Patriarchy and the Case for Socialist Feminism*. Monthly Review Press, New York.
Hartmann H (1981) The unhappy marriage of Marxism and Feminism: towards a more progressive union. In Sargent L (ed.) *Women and Revolution*. Pluto, London, pp. 1–41.
Hearn J (1982) Notes on patriarchy, professionalisation and the semi-professions. *Sociology* **16**(2): 184–202.
Henwood M (1992) *Through a Glass Darkly: Community Care and Elderly People*. King's Fund Institute, London.
Henwood M (1993) Age discrimination in health care. In Johnson J and Slater M (eds) *Ageing and Later Life*. Sage, London, pp. 112–19.
Hershberger S L and D'Augelli A R (1995) The impact of victimisation on the mental health and suicidality of lesbian, gay and bisexual youths. *Developmental Psychology* **31**(1): 65–74.
Hillan E M (1993) Nursing dementing elderly people: ethical issues. *Journal of Advanced Nursing* **18**(12): 1889–94.
Hitchcock J M and Wilson H S (1992) Personal risking, lesbian self disclosure of sexual orientation to professional health care providers. *Nursing Research* May/June: 178–83.
Hochschild H (1983) *The Managed Heart*. University of California Press, Berkley, CA.
Holland J, Ramazanoglu C, Scott S, Sharpe S and Thompson R (1990) Sex, gender and power: young women's sexuality in the shadow of AIDS. *Sociology of Health and Illness* **12**(3): 336–50.
hooks B (1992) *Ain't I a Woman*. Pluto Press, London.
Hopton J (1995)User involvement in the education of mental health nurses: an evaluation of possibilities. *Critical Social Policy* **42**: 42–60.
Hoyes L, Jeffers, Lart R, Means R and Taylor M (1993) *User Empowerment and the Reform of Community Care*. School of Advanced Urban Studies Publications, Bristol.
Hughes B (1995) *Older People and Community Care*. Open University Press, Buckingham.
Hughes D (1988) When nurse knows best: some aspects of nurse/doctor interaction in a casualty department. *Sociology of Health and Illness* **10**(1): 1–22.
Hughes E (1956) The making of a physician. *Human Organisation* Winter: 21–5.
Hughes L (1990) Professionalising domesticity: a synthesis of selected nursing historiography. *Advanced Nursing Science* **12**(14): 25–31.
Hugman R (1991) *Power in Caring Professions*. Macmillan, Basingstoke.
Illich I (1977) *Limits to Medicine*. Penguin, Harmondsworth.
Irwin R (1992) Critical re-evaluation can overcome discrimination. Providing equal standards of care for homosexual patients. *Professional Nurse* 7(4): 435–8.

James K and Biley F (1989) Patient participation. *Nursing Standard* **18**(3): 32.
James N (1989) Emotional labour: skill and work in the social regulation of feelings. *Sociological Review* **37**: 15–41.
James N (1992) Care = organisation + physical labour + emotional labour. *Sociology of Health and Illness* **14**(4): 488–509.
James T, Harding I and Corbett K (1994) Biased care. *Nursing Times* **90**(51): 28–31.
James V and Gabe J (1996) *Health and the Sociology of Emotions*. Blackwell, Oxford.
Johnson J and Bytheway W (1993) Ageism: concept and definition. In Johnson J and Slater R (eds) *Ageing and Later Life*. Sage, London, pp. 200–6.
Johnson M (1990) Dependency and interdependency. In Bond S and Coleman P (eds) *Ageing in Society: An Introduction to Social Gerontology*. Sage, London, pp. 209–26.
Johnson M (1991) The meaning of old age. In Redfern S (ed.) *Nursing Elderly People*. Churchill Livingstone, Edinburgh, pp. 3–18.
Johnson T J (1972) *Professions and Power*. Macmillan, Basingstoke.
Jolley M (1989) The professionalisation of nursing: the uncertain path. In Jolley M and Allan P (eds) *Current Issues in Nursing*. Chapman & Hall, London, pp. 1–22.
Jones A (1988) Nothing gay about bereavement. *Nursing Times* **84**(23): 55–7.
Jones K (1972) *A History of the Mental Health Services*. Routledge & Kegan Paul, London.
Jones L C (1994) *The Social Context of Health and Health Work*. Macmillan, London.
Jury L (1993) *Guardian*, 28 July, p. 3. 'Shocking vendetta' against handicapped.
Katz F (1969) Nurses. In Etzioni A (ed.) *The Semi-Professions and their Organisation: Teachers, Nurses, Social Workers*. Free Press, New York, pp. 54–81.
Kelly L (1988) *Surviving Sexual Abuse*. Polity Press, Cambridge.
Kennedy P and Grey N (1997) High pressure areas. *Nursing Times* **93**(29): 26–31.
King's Fund (1995) *We Thought We Knew... Involving Patients in Nursing Practice*. King's Fund Nursing Development Programme, London.
King's Fund Panel (1989) *Intensive Care in the United Kingdom: Report from the King's Fund Panel*. King's Fund, London.
Koetting M E (1996) A group design for HIV negative gay men. *Social Work* **41**(4): 407–15.
Larsson S, Lestrange N, McLennan W and Latta L (1995) Fracture of the hip in elderly people. In Rowley D and Benedict C (eds) *Skeletal Trauma in Old Age*. Chapman & Hall, London, pp. 125–54.
Lawler J (1991) *Behind the Screens. Nursing Somology and the Problems of the Body*. Churchill Livingstone, Melbourne.

LeGrand J and Bartlett W (eds) (1993) *Quasi-Markets and Social Policy*. Macmillan, Basingstoke.
Ley P and Spelman M (1967) *Communications with the Patient*. Saples Press, London.
Limpinnian M (1991) A community nursing home as an alternative to hospital care: Are we following the right route? Unpublished MSc dissertation, School of Advanced Urban Studies, University of Bristol.
Lindow V (1993) A vision for the future. In Beresford P and Harding T (eds) *A Challenge to Change: Practical Experiences of Building User-led Services*. National Institute for Social Workers, London.
Lindow V and Morris J (1995) *Service User Involvement*. Joseph Rowntree Foundation, York.
Lorber J (1991) Dismantling Noah's Ark. In Lorber J and Farrell S (eds) *The Social Construction of Gender*. Sage, London.
Lorbiecki A (1995) Clinicians as managers: conveyance or collision. In Soothill K, Mackay L and Webb C (eds) *Interprofessional Relations in Health Care*. Edward Arnold, London, pp. 88–106.
Luker K A, Beaver K, Leinster S J and Owens R G (1993) Preferences for information and decision making in women newly diagnosed with breast cancer: final report. Unpublished Report for the Cancer Relief Macmillan Fund.
Luker K A, Beaver K, Leinster S J and Owens R G (1996) Information needs and sources of information for women with breast cancer: a follow-up study. *Journal of Advanced Nursing* **23**: 487–95.
Lukes S (1974) *Power: A Radical View*. Macmillan, Basingstoke.
Lupton D (1996) Your life in their hands. In James V and Gabe J (eds) *Health and the Sociology of Emotions*. Blackwell, Oxford, pp. 157–72.
Lyotard J (1984) *The Postmodern Condition: A Report on Knowledge*. Manchester University Press, Manchester.
Maben J and Macleod Clark J (1997) The impact of Project 2000. *Nursing Times* **93**(35): 55–8.
McArdle J M C, George W D, McArdle C S *et al.* (1996) Psychological support for patients undergoing breast cancer surgery: a randomised study. *British Medical Journal* **312**: 813–17.
McDougal J (1993) Therapeutic issues with gay and lesbian elders. *Clinical Gerontologist* **14**(1): 45–57.
Mackay L (1989) *Nursing a Problem*. Open University Press, Buckingham.
Mackay L (1995) The patient as pawn in interprofessional relationships. In Soothill K, Mackay L and Webb C (eds) *Interprofessional Relations in Health Care*. Edward Arnold, London, pp. 349–60.
MacKinnon C (1989) *Towards a Feminist Theory of the State*. Harvard University Press, Cambridge, MA.
McLeod E (1995) Patients in interprofessional practice. In Soothill K, Mackay L and Webb C (eds) *Interprofessional Relations in Health Care*. Edward Arnold, London, pp. 332–48.

Macleod M (1994) 'It's the little things that count': the hidden complexity of everyday clinical nursing practice. *Journal of Clinical Nursing* **3**(6): 361–8.
McMillan I (1997) Refuge reaching out. *Nursing Standard* **11**(39): 26–7.
MacNay L (1994) *Foucault – A Critical Introduction*. Polity Press, Cambridge.
Malin N and Teasdale K (1991) Caring versus empowerment: considerations for nursing practice. *Journal of Advanced Nursing* **16**: 657–62.
Manthey M (1980) *The Practice of Primary Nursing*. Blackwell, Oxford.
Marks L (1994) *Seamless Care or Patchwork Quilt? Discharging Patients From Acute Hospital Care*. King's Fund Institute, London.
Marks-Maran D J and Pope B M (1985) *Breast Cancer Nursing and Counselling*. Blackwell, Oxford.
May C (1991) Affective neutrality and involvement in nurse–patient relationships: perceptions of appropriate behaviour among nurses in acute medical and surgical wards. *Journal of Advanced Nursing* **16**: 552–8.
May C (1992a) Individualised care? Power and subjectivity in therapeutic relations. *Sociology* **26**: 589–602.
May C (1992b) Nursing work, nurses' knowledge and the subjectification of the patient. *Sociology of Health and Illness* **14**: 472–87.
Means R and Smith R (1994) *Community Care: Policy and Practice*. Macmillan, Basingstoke.
Means R, Hoyes L, Lart R and Taylor M (1994) Quasi-markets and community care: towards user empowerment? In Bartlett W, Propper C, Wilson D and LeGrand J (eds) *Quasi-Markets in the Welfare State*. School of Advanced Urban Studies Publications, Bristol.
Meeuwesen L, Schaap C and Vander Staak C (1991) Verbal analysis of doctor–patient communication. *Social Science and Medicine* **32**: 1143–50.
Melia K (1987) *Learning and Working: The Occupational Socialisation of Nurses*. Tavistock, London.
Memmi A (1965) *The Coloniser and the Colonised*. Orion Press, New York.
Menzies I (1970) *The Functioning of Social Systems as a Defense Against Anxiety*. Tavistock, London.
Merton R K (1957) Some preliminaries to a sociology of medical education. In Merton R K, Reader G and Kendall P L (eds) *The Student Physician*. Harvard University Press, Cambridge, MA.
Merquior J (1991) *Foucault*. Fontana, London.
Meutzel P-A (1988) Therapeutic nursing. In Pearson A (ed.) *Primary Nursing: Nursing in the Burford and Oxford Nursing Development Units*. Chapman & Hall, London, pp. 89–116.
Miers M (1990) Developing skills in decision making. *Nursing Times* **86**(30): 32–3.
Miliband R (1969) *The State in Capitalist Society*. Weidenfeld & Nicolson, London.

Miller A (1989) Theory to practice: implementation in the clinical setting. In Jolley M and Allan P (eds) *Current Issues in Nursing*. Chapman & Hall, London, pp. 47–66.
Millet K (1970) *Sexual Politics*. Doubleday, New York.
Mills C W (1956) *The Power Elite*. Oxford University Press, Oxford.
MIND (1992)*The MIND Guide to Advocacy in Mental Health: Empowerment in Action*. MIND, London.
Mitchell G (1989) Empowerment and opportunity. *Social Work Today* **20** (27): 14.
Morrall P (1996) Clinical sociology and the empowerment of clients. *Mental Health Nursing* **16**(3): 24–7.
Morris J (1993) Working together: the expression of choice. In Beresford P and Harding T (eds) *Practical Experiences of Building User-led Services: A Challenge to Change*. National Institute for Social Work, London.
Morris J and Royle G J (1988) Offering patients a choice of surgery for early breast cancer: a reduction in anxiety and depression in patients and their husbands. *Social Science and Medicine* **26**(6): 583–85.
Mosca G (1939) *The Ruling Class*. McGraw-Hill, New York.
Muff J (1982) Handmaiden, battle-axe, whore: an exploration into the fantasies, myths and stereotypes about nurses. In Muff J (ed.) *Socialization, Sexism and Stereotyping: Women's Issues in Nursing*. Waveland, Prospect Heights, IL, pp. 113–56.
Mullender A and Ward D (1991) *Self-directed Groupwork: Users Take Action for Empowerment*. Whiting & Birch, London.
National Boards for England and Wales (1986) *Syllabus of Training 1982: Professional Register – Part 3 (Registered Mental Nurse)*. English National Board, London.
Nelson J A (1997) Gay, lesbian and bisexual adolescents: providing esteem enhancing care to a battered population. *Nurse Practitioner* **22**(2): 94–103.
Ness M and Ryrie I (1997) A change for the better. *Nursing Times* **93**(23): 36–9.
Nettleton S (1992) *Power, Pain and Dentistry*. Open University Press, Buckingham.
Nettleton S (1995) From the hospital to community care: Foucauldian analyses. In Heyman B (ed.) *Researching User Perspectives in Community Health Care*. Chapman & Hall, London, pp. 232–43.
Newall J (1996) Power in Project 2000 nursing. Unpublished dissertation towards MSc in Social Research, University of Bath.
NHS Executive (1996) *A Patient's Charter: Services for Children and Young People*. NHSE, London.
Oakley A (1972) *Sex, Gender and Society*. Temple Smith, London.
Oakley A (1984) The importance of being a nurse. *Nursing Times* **80**(50): 24–7.
O'Brien J (1981) *The Principle of Normalisation: A Foundation for Effective Services* (adapted by Tyne A). Campaign for Mentally Handicapped People, London.

Office of Health Economics (1995) *Compendium of Health Statistics*. Office of Health Economics, London.
Office for National Statistics (1997) *Social Trends 27*. HMSO, London.
Oliver M (1990) *The Politics of Disablement*. Macmillan, London.
Opie A (1997) Thinking teams, thinking clients: issues of discourse and representation in the work of health care teams. *Sociology of Health and Illness* **19**(3): 259–80.
Pareto V (1963) *A Treatise on General Sociology*. Edited by Livingston A, Dover Publications, New York.
Parkin F (1979) *Marxism and Class Theory: A Bourgeois Critique*. Tavistock, London.
Parry N and Parry J (1976) *The Rise of the Medical Profession*. Croom Helm, London.
Parsons E (1994) Technology and the nursing dilemma. A sociological analysis of modernism and post modernism in intensive care units. In Millar B and Burnard P (eds) *Critical Care Nursing*. Baillière Tindall, London, pp. 290–312.
Parsons T (1951) *The Social System*. Free Press, New York.
Pearson A (1988) Primary nursing. In Pearson A, *Primary Nursing: Nursing in the Burford and Oxford Nursing Development Units*. Chapman & Hall, London, pp. 1–39.
Pembrey S (1985) A framework for care. *Nursing Times*, 11 December: 47–9.
Penn K (1994) Patient advocacy in palliative care. *British Journal of Nursing* **3**(1): 40–2.
Peplau H (1969) Professional closeness. *Nursing Forum* **8**(4): 342–60.
Perry A (1993) A sociologist's view: the handmaiden's theory. In Jolley M and Brykczynska G (eds) *Nursing – Its Hidden Agendas*. Edward Arnold, London.
Phillips A (1987) *Divided Loyalties*. Virago, London.
Phillipson P (1993) Approaches to advocacy. In Johnson J and Slater R (eds) *Ageing and Later Life*. Sage, London, pp. 181–7.
Philpot T (1993) *Whose assessment is it anyway?* Search March, Joseph Rowntree Foundation, York.
Philpot T (1994) *Managing to Listen: A Guide to User Involvement for Mental Health Service Managers*. King's Fund, London.
Phoenix NHS Trust and County of Avon Social Services (1995) *Shared Action Planning*. Phoenix NHS Trust, Bristol.
Platzer H (1990) Sexual orientation: improving care. *Nursing Standard* **4**(38): 38–9.
Pole J (1996) Years of living dangerously. *Guardian*, March 6: 7.
Porter S (1991) A participant observation study of power relations between nurses and doctors in a general hospital. *Journal of Advanced Nursing* **16**: 728–35.
Porter S (1995a) Northern nursing: the limits of idealism. *Irish Journal of Sociology* **5**: 22–42.
Porter S (1995b) *Nursing's Relationship with Medicine*. Avebury, Aldershot.

Porter S (1996) Contra-Foucault: soldiers, nurses and power. *Sociology* **30**(1): 59–78.
Porter S (1998) *Social Theory and Nursing Practice*. Macmillan, Basingstoke.
Poulantzas N (1978) *State, Power, Socialism*. New Left Books, London.
Prior L (1991) Community versus hospital care: the crisis in psychiatric provision. *Social Science and Medicine* **32**(4): 483–9.
Rabinow P (ed.) (1991) *The Foucault Reader. An Introduction to Foucault's Thought*. Penguin, London.
Ranade W (1994) *A Future for the NHS? Health Care in the 1990s*. Longman, London.
Razmanoglu C (1989) *Feminism and the Contradictions of Oppression*. Routledge, London.
Redfern S (1991) Continuing care in the long-stay settings. In Redfern S (ed.) *Nursing Elderly People*. Churchill Livingstone, Edinburgh, pp. 497–518.
Reid Y and Garety P (1996) A hostel ward for new long stay patients: sixteen years progress. *Journal of Mental Health* **5**(1): 77–89.
Rich A (1977) *Of Woman Born: Motherhood as Experience and Institution*. Virago, London.
Rich A (1986) *Blood, Bread and Poetry. Selected Prose 1979–1985*. Virago, London.
Riska E and Wegar K (1993) Women physicians: a new force in medicine? In Riska E and Wegar K (eds) *Gender, Work and Medicine*. Sage, London, pp. 77–93.
Roberts S (1983) Oppressed group behaviour: implications for nursing. *Advances in Nursing Science* **5**(4): 21–30.
Roberts S J and Sorensen L (1995) Lesbian healthcare: a review and recommendations for health promotion in primary care settings. *Nurse Practitioner* **20**(6): 42–7.
Robinson K (1992) The nursing workforce: aspects of inequality. In Robinson J, Gray A and Elkan R (eds) *Policy Issues in Nursing*. Open University Press, Buckingham.
Rogers A, Pilgrim D and Lacey R (1993) *Experiencing Psychiatry: Users' Views of Services*. MIND, London.
Rose P (1993) Out in the open. *Nursing Times* **89**(30): 50–2.
Royal College of Nursing (1994a) Nursing care for gay men and lesbians. *Nursing Standard* **8**(48): 32.
Royal College of Nursing (1994b) *Standards of Care: Breast Cancer Nursing*. London, Royal College of Nursing.
Ryan J and Thomas F (1980) *The Politics of Mental Handicap*. Penguin, Harmondsworth.
Sainsbury Centre for Mental Health (1997) *Pulling Together: The Future Roles and Training of Mental Health Workforce*. Sainsbury Centre for Mental Health, London.
Sallah D (1996) Alternatives to seclusion. In Sandford T and Gournay K (eds) *Perspectives in Mental Health Nursing*. Baillière Tindall, London.

Salmon B (1968) *Report of the Committee on Senior Nurse Staff Structure*. HMSO, London.
Salsberry P J (1993) Assuming responsibility for one's health. An analysis of a key assumption in nursing's agenda for health care reform. *Nursing Outlook* **41**(5): 212–16.
Salvage J (1985) *The Politics of Nursing*. Heinemann, Oxford.
Salvage J (1992) The new nursing: empowering patients or empowering nurses? In Robinson J, Gray A and Elkan R (eds) *Policy Issues in Nursing*. Open University Press, Buckingham.
Savage J (1995) *Nursing Intimacy. An Ethnographic Approach to Nurse Patient Interaction*. Scutari Press, London.
Scandlyn J (1988) Social aspects of AIDS. *Orthopaedic Nursing* 7(5): 26–32.
Schön D (1983) *The Reflective Practitioner: How Professionals Think in Action*. Temple Smith, London.
Sheehan A (1996) Mental health nursing development units. In Sandford T and Gournay K (eds) *Perspectives in Mental Health Nursing*. Baillière Tindall, London, pp. 17–30.
Shepherd G, Muijen M, Dean R and Cosney M (1996) Residential care in hospital and in the community – quality of care and quality of life. *British Journal of Psychiatry* **168**: 446–56.
Simmons S and Brooker C (1986) Community psychiatric nursing: a social perspective. Heinemann, London.
Slevin M L, Plant H, Lynch D, Drinkwater J and Gregory W M (1988) Who should measure the quality of life, the doctor or the patient? *British Journal of Cancer* **57**: 109–12.
Slevin M L, Stubbs L, Plant H J *et al.* (1990) Attitudes to chemotherapy: comparing views of patients with cancer with those of doctors, nurses and general public. *British Medical Journal* **300**(2): 1458–60.
Smith G B (1993) Homophobia and attitudes to gay men and lesbians by psychiatric nurses. *Archives of Psychiatric Nursing* **VII**(6): 377–84.
Smith P (1988) The emotional labour of nursing. *Nursing Times* **84**(44): 50–1.
Smith P (1992) *The Emotional Labour of Nursing*. Macmillan, Basingstoke.
SSRU (Social Science Research Unit) (1994) *Women's Views of Breast Cancer Treatment and Research*. Institute of Education, London.
Stacey J (1997) Feminist Theory: capital F, capital T. In Robinson V and Richardson D (eds) *Introducing Women's Studies*, 2nd edn. Macmillan, Basingstoke, pp. 54–76.
Stacey M (1992) *Regulating British Medicine: The General Medical Council*. Wiley, Chichester.
Stanworth M (ed.) (1987) *Reproductive Technologies: Gender, Motherhood and Medicine*. Polity Press, Cambridge.
Stein L (1967) The doctor–nurse game. *Archives of General Psychiatry* **16**: 699–703.

Stein L (1978) The doctor–nurse game. In Dingwall R and McIntosh J (eds) *Readings in the Sociology of Nursing*. Churchill Livingstone, Edinburgh, pp. 107–17.
Stevens P E (1992) Lesbian health care research: a review of the literature from 1970–1990. *Health Care for Women International* **13**(2): 91–120.
Stevens P E (1994) Lesbians' health related experiences of care and non care. *Western Journal of Nursing Research* **16**(6): 639–59.
Stevens P E (1995) Structural and interpersonal impact of heterosexual assumptions on lesbian health care clients. *Nursing Research* **44**(1): 25–30.
Stevens P E and Hall J M (1988) Stigma, health beliefs and experiences with health care in lesbian women. *Image, Journal of Nursing Scholarship* **20**(2): 69–73.
Stevenson O and Parsloe P (1993) *Community Care and Empowerment*. Joseph Rowntree Foundation, York.
Strauss A (1978) *Negotiations: Varieties, Contexts, Processes and Social Order.* Jossey-Bass, London.
Strong P (1978) *The Ceremonial Order of the Clinic*. Routledge & Kegan Paul, London.
Sutherland G (1984) *Ability, Merit and Measurement*. Macmillan, Basingstoke.
Sutherland H J, Llewellyn-Thomas H A, Lockwood G A, Tritchler D L and Till J E (1989) Cancer patients: their desire for information and participation in treatment decisions. *Journal of the Royal Society of Medicine* **82**: 260–3.
Svensson R (1996) The interplay between doctors and nurses – a negotiated order perspective. *Sociology of Health and Illness* **18**: 379–98.
Synoground S G and Kellmer-Langan D (1991) Nursing students' attitudes towards AIDS. *Nurse Education Today* **11**(3): 200–6.
Taylor B A and Remafedi G (1993) Youth coping with sexual orientation issues. *Journal of School Nursing* **9**(2): 26–37.
Taylor I and Robertson A (1994) The health needs of gay men: a discussion of the literature and implications for nursing. *Journal of Advanced Nursing* **20**: 560–6.
Taylor M, Hoyes L, Lart R and Means R (1992) *User Empowerment in Community Care: Unravelling the Issues*. School of Advanced Urban Studies Publications, Bristol.
Thomas B, Hardy S and Cutting P (eds) (1997) *Stuart and Sundeen's Mental Health Nursing: Principles and Practice*. C V Mosby, London.
Thompson K (ed.) (1984) *Work Employment and Unemployment*. Open University Press, Buckingham.
Thompson L (1994) Role of the breast care nurse at the point of diagnosis. Speech at the Royal College of Nursing Breast Care Nursing Society Conference 1993. Reported in *Breast Care Nursing* Winter 1993/4: 3.
Thomson M (1992) Community care and control of mental defectives in interwar Britain. Paper given to the SSHM Annual Conference Communities, Caring and Institutions.

Thornton C (1997) Meeting the health care needs of people with learning disabilities. *Nursing Times* **93**(20): 52–4.
Thornton H (1993) Whose interests: patient's or researcher's? *Bulletin of Medical Ethics* **93**: 13–19.
Tong R (1992) *Feminist Thought: A Comprehensive Introduction*. Routledge, London.
Torensen M (1995) Sexual healing. *Emergency Nurse* **3**(1): 4–5.
Townsend P (1986) Ageism and social policy. In Phillipson C and Walker A (eds) *Ageing and Social Policy: A Critical Assessment*. Gower, Aldershot, pp. 15–44.
Trippet S E (1994) Lesbians' mental health concerns. *Health Care for Women International* **15**: 317–23.
Turner B (1987) *Medical Power and Social Knowledge*. Sage, London.
United Kingdom Central Council for Nursing, Midwifery and Health Visiting (1986) *Project 2000: A new preparation for practice*. UKCC/London University Press, London.
United Kingdom Central Council for Nursing, Midwifery and Health Visiting (1989) *Exercising Accountability*. UKCC/London University Press, London.
United Kingdom Central Council for Nursing, Midwifery and Health Visiting (1992a) *The Scope of Professional Practice*. UKCC/London University Press, London.
United Kingdom Central Council For Nursing, Midwifery and Health Visiting (1992b) *Code of Conduct for the Nurse, Midwife and Health Visitor*, 3rd edn. UKCC/London University Press, London.
United Kingdom Central Council for Nursing, Midwifery and Health Visiting (1996) *Guidelines for Professional Practice*. UKCC/London University Press, London.
Wadler J (1992) *My Breast: One Woman's Cancer Story*. Womens' Press/Wadsworth, London.
Walby S (1990) *Theorising Patriarchy*. Blackwell, Oxford.
Walby S, Greenwell J, Mackay L and Soothill K (1994) *Medicine and Nursing: Professions in a Changing Health Service*. Sage, London.
Walker A (1990) Poverty and inequality in old age. In Bond S and Calman P (eds) *Ageing in Society: An Introduction to Social Gerontology*. London, Sage, pp. 229–49.
Wallcraft C (1994) Empowering, empowerment, professionals and self advocacy projects. *Mental Health Nursing* **14**(2): 6–7.
Walsh M and Ford P (1989) It can't hurt that much. *Nursing Times* **85**(42): 35–8.
Walters T (1991) Modern death: taboo or not taboo? *Sociology* **25**(2): 293–310.
Watkins S and Wilson E (1997) Establishing a public health nursing project. *Nursing Standard* **11**(36): 44–8.
Watson J C (1985) *HumanSciences and Human Care: A Theory of Nursing*. Appleton Crofts, Norwalk, CT.

Webb C and Askham J (1987) Nurses' knowledge and attitudes about sexuality in health care – a review of the literature. *Nurse Education Today* **7**: 75–87.

Weber M (1948) *From Max Weber: Essays in Sociology* (eds and trans H H Gerth and C Wright Mills). Routledge & Kegan Paul, London.

Weber M (1968) *Economy and Society*, vol. 2. Bedminster Press, New York.

Weiler K (1988) *Women Teaching for Change*. Bergin and Garvey, New York.

Wertheimer A (1993) *Speaking Out: Citizen Advocacy and Older People*. Centre for Policy on Ageing, London.

Wheeler S (1995) Child abuse: the health perspective. In Kingston P and Penhale B (eds) *Family Violence and the Caring Professions*. Macmillan, Basingstoke, pp. 50–76.

Wickler D (1987) Personal responsibility for illness. In Van De Veer D and Regan T (eds) *Health Care Ethics*. Temple University Press, Philadelphia.

Wilkinson P (1992) The influence of high technology care on patients, relatives and their nurses. *Intensive and Critical Care Nursing* **8**(4): 194–8.

Willis P (1977) *Learning to Labour*. Gower, London.

Witz A (1992) *Professions and Patriarchy*. Routledge, London.

Witz A and Savage M (1992) The gender of organisation. In Witz A and Savage M (eds) *Gender and Bureaucracy*. Blackwell, Oxford.

Wolf Z R (1986a) Nurses' work: the sacred and the profane. *Holistic Nursing Practice* **1**(1): 29–35.

Wolf Z R (1986b) *Nursing Rituals in an Adult Acute Care Hospital: An Ethnography*. University of Pennsylvania School of Nursing, University Microfilms, Ann Arbor, MI.

Wolf Z R (1996) Bowel management and nursing's hidden work. *Nursing Times* **92**(21): 26–8.

Woodhouse S (1990) Why have medicine rounds? *Paediatric Nursing* **2**(10): 9–11.

Wright D and Digby A (eds) (1996) *From Idiocy to Mental Deficiency: Historical Perspective on People with Learning Difficulties*. Routledge, London.

Wright S G (1986) *Building and Using a Model of Nursing*. Edward Arnold, Sevenoaks.

Wright S (1995) *Work from Nursing Development Units: We Thought We Knew... Involving Patients in Nursing Practice: An Executive Summary*. King's Fund, London.

Zaretsky E (1976) *Capitalism, the Family and Personal Life*. Pluto Press, London.

Zeidenstein L (1990) Gynaecological and child bearing needs of lesbians. *Journal of Nurse Midwifery* **35**(1): 10–18.

Zola I (1975) In the name of health and illness: on some practical consequences of medical influence. *Social Science and Medicine* **9**: 83–7.

Name Index

Subject Index